MW00659077

An Integrative Approach

to Healing Chronic Illness:

Revealing the Root Causes

of Modern Disease

By Richard Brightheart, M.Ac., L.Ac., L.M.P.

Center for Energetic Healing

An Integrative Approach to Healing Chronic Illness: Revealing the Root Causes of Modern Disease

By Richard Brightheart, M.Ac., L.Ac., L.M.P.

Printed by: Gorham Printing
3718 Mahoney Drive
Centralia, WA 98531

All rights reserved. No part of this book may be reproduced, stored in a retrieval system or transmitted, in any form or by any means, electronic, mechanical, photocopying, recording or otherwise, without the prior written permission of the author, except for brief quotations in a review.

Cover design: Heather Crank
Editor: Rita R. Robison

Printed in the United States of America
ISBN 0-9798770-0-8   ISBN13 978-0-9798770-0-1

Copyright © 2007 by Richard Brightheart, M.Ac., L.Ac., L.M.P.
Second Edition 2009
Third Edition 2010
Fourth Edition 2017

Disclaimer: The information in this book is intended for education, entertainment, research and information purposes only. This information is not intended to be used to diagnose, prescribe or replace proper medical treatment. Nutritional protocols and information described in the book are not intended to treat, cure, diagnose, mitigate or prevent any disease.

For information: Visit the Healing Energy Approach website at www.richbrightheart.com for updated nutritional information, environmental and nutritional sensitivities news, and the latest research on emerging pathogenic influences causing illness.

Contents

Introduction

Illness itself has drastically changed in the last twenty years. In the last ten years, I have seen more and more chronic illness in my practice. The environment for the creation of illness has become much more complex. The playing field has shifted with new rules. Hybrid toxins and pathogens are infiltrating our interior environment with very little resistance.

Our soil, water and poor air quality are helping to create a multitude of new diseases. New mutated forms of viruses and bacteria are not only surviving whatever antibiotic we use, they are becoming stronger and more resistant in the process. Besides human immunodeficiency virus (HIV), there are a number of other types of stealth pathogens such as mycoplasmas, the spirochete *Borrelia burgdorferi* as in Lyme disease, mycobacterium and other cell wall deficient and intracellular pathogenic forms that are now creating an enormous amount of chronic illness inside much of our unknowing population. Our air, soil, food, water and oceans are now so polluted that most individuals have huge amounts of toxic chemicals coexisting within their own cells. Most of these poisons did not exist in the past. Toxic drug residues are leaking into our drinking water and oceans that may cause unimaginable illnesses in the future. Electromagnetic smog is becoming a real health issue, which may bring on a whole host of new created illnesses.

These environmental shifts are creating a wide range of infectious and toxic-based diseases that are at the core of much of the chronic inflammatory and deteriorating conditions that are plaguing so many of us. Our immune systems are being challenged daily due to stress, pollution and infestation of these hybrid forms of pathogens. Humans were not designed to be hosts for these types of invaders and toxic substances. We are literally being poisoned and taken over at the cellular level. Cancer, heart disease, diabetes, fibromyalgia, multiple sclerosis, arthritis, irritable bowel syndrome/Crohn's disease, chronic fatigue syndrome, and countless other chronic inflammatory and autoimmune diseases and syndromes are at an all-time high. Many of these illnesses did not exist just a few decades ago.

An Integrative Approach to Healing Chronic Illness: Revealing the Root Causes of Modern Disease is the first and only book that pulls the curtain aside, revealing the scientific truth behind much of the causative factors underlying these modern-day illnesses that are being ignored by mainstream medicine. This book is filled with scientific, factual and clinically based evidence as supportive proof for why these changes have come about in our lifetime. People can now understand the root causes of many of these seemingly mysterious diseases and have some of the latest information on current treatment options, as well as therapeutically based nutritional formulas.

Traditional medicine has little understanding and few answers for these chronic illnesses, except to treat the symptoms with drugs or perform surgery, once they have reached a diseased state. There are many misconceptions in the health arena, perpetuated by the manner in which health care is presented. The media have a tremendous amount of influence on how the public perceives illness and subsequent treatment options (Moynihan, 2005). They have been promoting certain ideals that support this way of thinking for years. These ideas have been so ingrained into our society that they block many people from their own ability to think for themselves. America spends much more money on health care compared to other countries; however, this has not translated to better overall health. The United States ranks thirty-seventh in overall quality of health care despite the fact that we spend twice the cost per capita compared with other developed nations, according to the World Health Organization (Garritano, January 10, 2007).

Medical care expenditures are so high because traditional medicine looks at the disease process and emphasizes labeling various symptoms and effects into a named disease or syndrome. Medical schools teach doctors how to become experts on labeling disease, and which drugs should be used in order to best manage the disease category in which people are placed. Success in this scenario is judged by how well a doctor can suppress a patient's symptoms, in relationship to how many side effects are subsequently developed from the drugs that they are taking. Strong educational influences from the drug industry perpetuate this way of thinking. The modern term for this way of practicing medicine is called "disease management." It seldom addresses the causative factors behind the labeled disease, but perpetuates the concept that treating illness from a symptomatic perspective is not only acceptable, but is considered state-of-the-art medicine. The two most important things that a doctor should know are: what is causing a patient's illness and how to get rid of it. Everything else is just a label, and nothing more.

An Integrative Approach to Healing Chronic Illness: Revealing the Root Causes of Modern Disease examines why illness and treatment options are represented in their present form by the medical profession, and served up on a silver platter by the media. Readers will understand why illness as defined by traditional medicine is just an effect, and they will learn about what really causes illness. *An Integrative Approach to Healing Chronic Illness* breaks down diseases and syndromes into their basic root causes.

My original intention was to write individual papers explaining the causes of various illnesses that may be associated with my patients' symptoms, since my practice had become too busy to explain fairly complicated scenarios. By handing my patients a paper, they could get all the information they needed to understand the causes of their illness. This seemed to work well, as I could devote extra time to other patients. It was especially helpful early in their healing process. As I was writing piece after piece, I began to realize that everyone, not just my patients, should be aware of this information, so they as well could fully understand their illness. I decided writing a book would help people make better choices about their own health care.

I also believe *An Integrative Approach to Healing Chronic Illness: Revealing the Root Causes of Modern Disease* can be of great benefit to health care practitioners who are willing to learn about these concepts in order to help their patients get well.

The book's content comes from more than thirty years of research, education, clinical experience and practical application. My idea of what causes illness has evolved over this time. I am open to learning and researching any new healing modality, or idea that comes my way. I am not invested in a certain modality, corporation or way of looking at disease. My education, research and clinical results have become my belief system. My thirty plus years in private practice, as well as countless hours of research, have been consumed with my passion for finding the actual cause of many illnesses. My clinical work has reflected this basic idea. I have worked with thousands of patients, helping to heal many from supposedly incurable illnesses.

The labeling of a certain disease process is just a label. All illness is merely an effect and nothing more. Once the cause is identified and treated, then the effect is past tense, and so is the named disease. Most illness breaks down to three or four basic physical causes. Because people are told that they have fibromyalgia (inflammation of the muscle fibers) does nothing to solve the problem. They have a labeled disease with a complicated name, which only doctors fully understand. Lay people are at the medical community's mercy. This diagnosis can feel intimidating, especially when a health care professional says that nothing can be done, because no one knows what causes it or how to cure it. Remember that it is still most people's perception that the doctor is the authority on disease. Millions of intelligent people subscribe to these types of labels, because they are taught not to question medical authority. Many feel overwhelmed with the responsibility of having to take charge of their own health care. They want someone else to do it for them. They do little or none of their own investigating and searching for answers. They assume that if the medical experts have no answer or cure, then why would anyone else? If there were an answer, their doctor would surely know. Patients are left with little hope, and often do exactly what their doctor tells them. They end up owning their labeled disease by suffering needlessly, or at best managing the symptoms with drugs, without any hope for a cure. They bought the "labeled program" and are convinced they must live with the illness.

Patients who question their doctors and do their own research by reading, exploring the Internet and getting opinions from other types of health care practitioners have far better results than patients who do little or nothing, and say yes to whatever their doctors suggest. Viewing a wealth of information from a wide range of perspectives gives people the ability to be knowledgeable and objective in whatever form of treatment they decide to undertake. I want to emphasize that it is patients who should be in charge of their treatment after all the facts are in. Illness does not happen by accident; it always has a cause and effect. Learning this is the first step on the path to becoming well again.

Notes

Garritano, Joanna, M.D. "U.S. Health Care Puts Profit Over People," *Seattle Post-Intelligencer*, January 10, 2007.

Moynihan, Ray and Alan Cassels. *Selling Sickness: How the World's Biggest Pharmaceutical Companies Are Turning Us All Into Patients*. New York: Nation Books, 2005.

References

Abramson, John, M.D. *Overdosed America: The Broken Promise of American Medicine*. New York: Harper Perennial, 2005.

Dvonch, Louis, M.D., and Russell Dvonch. *The Heart Attack Germ: Prevent Strokes, Heart Attacks, and the Symptoms of Alzheimer's by Protecting Yourself From the Infections and Inflammation of Cardiovascular Disease*. New York: Writer's Showcase, 2003.

Nicolson, Garth L., Ph.D. "Chronic Fatigue Illnesses," The Institute for Molecular Medicine, Accessed June 26, 2005.
www.immed.org/illness/infectious_disease_research.html

Nicolson, Garth L., Ph.D. "Autoimmune Illnesses and Degenerative Diseases," The Institute for Molecular Medicine, Accessed June 26, 2005. www.immed.org/illness/fatigue_autoimmune_illness_research.html

Pugh, Tony. "Mediocre Doctoring the Norm," *The Denver Post*, March 18, 2006.

Siegel, Marc, M.D. "Who's in Charge? It's Your Care. Take Control of It, Recommends One Physician," *The Washington Post*, July 11, 2006.

Sinha, Gunjan. "Gulf War Illness: Psychological?" *Popular Science*, April 1999.

Chapter 1: Traditional and Nontraditional Approaches

Seeing thousands of patients in more than a thirty-year span has changed my views about how I perceive illness. During the 1980s taking supplements was popular. I thought that taking the best quality vitamins and eating the highest quality food, coupled with proper detoxification, was the right path to get well and protect myself from chronic illness.

Alternative medicine

Knowledge in the alternative medicine world has changed drastically since the 1980s. This is especially true in the category of bioenergetic medicine. This form of healing can make some of the biggest changes in one's health. Bioenergetic therapies have evolved as new methods have been discovered that have greatly enhanced what can be done for a patient. Many advanced nutritional formulas and herbal remedies have improved as well. Because of these advances, I can look at patients from many diverse angles to see what pieces of the puzzle are out of place and actually have the knowledge and tools to assist them in their healing process.

Criteria for practitioners

A doctor or health care practitioner needs to have two very important criteria in his toolbox in order to be an effective healer. The first is that he must be very knowledgeable about how the body functions and must have a strong educational background in anatomy and physiology. Secondly, the doctor needs to have a full understanding of what is actually causing the symptoms.

Traditional medicine

This is where it starts to get difficult, because traditional medical thinking and medical schools do not fully comprehend this basic premise. The medical establishment may teach tremendous amounts of knowledge about the body in terms of structure and function, but it fails to understand what actually causes many illnesses. It is a fact that universities of traditional medicine are greatly influenced by the pharmaceutical industry; they help to fund medical schools and their research. Therefore, they have a major stake in what type of education is taught, which in turn dictates the course of treatment to be determined by the health care professional.

The answer almost always involves drug therapy. The problem with this way of thinking is that, for the most part, drugs do not cure disease, but rather suppress the underlying problem by focusing on symptomatology. Practitioners leave traditional medical universities with this mindset, never questioning that their expensive education has not addressed the two most important questions, "What causes illness, and how to cure it?" Common sense tells us that this should be the main focus of a medical education. Most doctors have become experts in pharmacology and "disease management," instead of specialists in curing illness.

The big picture

When a health care practitioner sees a new patient who has had chronic symptoms for some time, the practitioner must understand that the patient probably has several underlying dysfunctions that are causing the symptoms. The health care practitioner has to look at the big picture. How many pieces of the puzzle are present? How are those pieces affecting their symptomatology, along with their overall picture of health? It can be complicated to determine where the practitioner needs to begin the diagnosis process.

There are few practitioners who have the training and expertise to understand the whole pattern. Looking at the big picture or whole person is not taught in the traditional medical schools; instead they tend to teach that the body is divided into separate compartments, which have little interaction with each other. This way of practicing medicine has a mindset in which you can stress one area of the body without understanding the long-term consequences and repercussions of corresponding areas of the body. This is simply not the way the body works. You cannot compartmentalize it in this manner. It must be viewed as a whole system, instead of a piece of a puzzle. This is why there are few doctors and practitioners practicing medicine that treat the root cause of illness. Most traditional doctors and practitioners tend to look at each patient from their training perspective. If the patient does not fit into the framework of her practitioner's thinking and training, then the patient probably will not improve much under the practitioner's care. The patient leaves feeling like no one understands her illness.

I firmly believe that if practitioners want to be effective healers, they must examine other options and be open minded to many ways of healing in order to assist patients in their healing process. Thinking out of the box is terrifying for some. However, looking back through history, it tells us that some of our greatest discoveries have come from nontraditional thinkers. Practitioners must venture out beyond the basic teachings, if they are going to be able to cure the diseases of our time. Practitioners need updated treatments that can effectively deal with the types of illnesses, which doctors and healers see on a regular basis.

The fact is many more potentially destructive health risks exist today than there were twenty years ago. I have seen much more chronic illness in my practice within the last ten years. The planet is becoming smaller every day, with our ability to board a plane and fly across the world in less than twenty-four hours. We are no longer isolated as we once were and this directly ties into the global causative factors for illness that have drastically changed the last two decades. Being healthy in our times is becoming a rarity, as illness is so common. The big difference now is that we do not die as often from many of these illnesses, but seem to be accustomed to accept poor health as a normal way of life.

References

Clemente, Carmine D., Ph.D. *Anatomy: A Regional Atlas of the Human Body*. Baltimore, Maryland: Urban and Schwarzenberg, 1987.

Deadman, Peter and Mazin Al-Khafaji. *A Manual of Acupuncture*. Vista, California: Eastland Press, 1998.

Giovanni, Maciocia. *The Practice of Chinese Medicine: The Treatment of Diseases With Acupuncture and Chinese Herbs*. London: Churchill Livingstone, 1994.

Oschman, James L., Ph.D. *Energy Medicine: The Scientific Basis*. London: Churchill Livingstone, 2000.

"Prescription Drug Deaths Take Leap in State Since '95," *The (Tacoma, Washington) News Tribune*, February 5, 2007.

Vander, Arthur J., M.D., James H. Sherman, Ph.D., and Dorothy S. Luciano, Ph.D. *Human Physiology*. New York: McGraw-Hill Inc., 1994.

Chapter 2: Energy Medicine

Energy medicine, the ability to work energetically at a cellular level with underlying causative agents, has existed for a long time. However, it has expanded in the types of energy techniques that are being practiced. Much progress has been made in the methods that have been developed. Energy medicine is a form of integrative medicine.

I have been practicing energy medicine for more than thirty years. You can make some of the biggest changes in your health by understanding how to use these types of modalities in therapeutic ways. Energy medicine differs greatly from biochemical medicine, which is the traditional medical model. Traditional medicine involves the manipulation of certain compounds, which force reactions to occur within the various body systems. It seems to have little regard or understanding for the delicate interactions between each organ system, especially when it involves long-term drug use.

The forms of energy medicine discussed here have existed for decades, some even for centuries.

Acupuncture

Acupuncture is probably the most well known of these therapies. It is an ancient healing art that has been practiced for more than three thousand years. Acupuncture uses the twelve meridians that run through the body, including most organs. Energy flow of qi runs through each meridian. There are also eight extra meridians that can be accessed by a skilled acupuncturist. A trained doctor of Chinese medicine can diagnose this qi in order to determine the health of the system. Meridians are best described as rivers of electrical current, as they can be electronically mapped. Any blockage along a meridian will cause a disruption of energy flow to the related organ that particular meridian runs through. This can lead to chronic organ dysfunction and eventual deterioration. Acupuncture points, which are positioned along each of these meridians, can have a huge effect in the way the energy or qi flows within that meridian, as well as associated ones. This is why acupuncture is such a powerful tool. Huge changes can happen instantaneously within that meridian and its associated organ, with the proper stimulation of certain points along its channel. The healthy flow of qi within each meridian has much to do with the overall health of the system. Stagnant, weak or blocked qi can lead to physical and emotional dysfunction on many levels. Chinese medicine understands that any imbalance in any one meridian may cause subsequent imbalance in another. This way of viewing the body is the basis of the yin and yang model of health.

Homeopathic medicine

Another form of energy medicine is homeopathic medicine. It existed long before drug companies began selling us on the idea that drugs and surgery are what we need. Homeopathic medicine uses diluted forms of substances given in small doses to treat problems. There are several forms or styles of homeopathic medicine being practiced. Homeopathics can be used for both acute and chronic problems. This can help with a host of diverse problems including allergies, emotional issues, detoxification, immune disorders, injuries and much more.

An example would be a diluted form of a substance such as wheat, which can be used to stimulate the immune system to help the body deal with it more effectively. Homeopathic medicine is a diluted form of energy that becomes stronger the more it is diluted. Most homeopathic remedies come in a tincture or pill form. Tinctures are usually made with alcohol. Water molecules within the body can store and carry energetic signals from homeopathic formulas that are conveying messages to the system. This messaging will interact with resonating cell receptors, thereby eliciting a systemic response.

Allergy elimination treatments

Allergy or sensitivity elimination treatments have generally been very successful because they can access this energetic system, which is like a computer. By changing the program within the circuitry, a new "program" can be written. The new program allows the body to not only tolerate substances that were once intolerable, but can allow the nutrients from those substances to be compatible with the current new program. This allows the body to absorb valuable nutrients that it once rejected, as well as reduce and/or eliminate unnecessary heightened immune responses. These energetic repatternings are usually permanent and often life changing.

Reiki, polarity therapy and therapeutic touch

Reiki, polarity therapy and therapeutic touch began to be used in the 1970s and 80s. They have several things in common such as touch and the movement of energy within the body. This transference of human energy through touch can have enormous therapeutic benefits within the body.

Reiki is probably the best known of all the energy therapies. During a Reiki session, the practitioner holds various areas throughout the body in a sequential order. There are thousands of trained Reiki practitioners across the country. People have had amazing results with this work, on both physical and emotional levels.

Polarity therapy is also a hands-on therapy that uses contact by the practitioner in order to facilitate balance through the body's electrical system. One of the first things I learned in polarity training is that the body is electrical in nature. It is composed primarily of water with positive and negatively charged ions suspended within this medium. Water is a great conductor of electricity and energy and can hold molecules in suspension. Molecules are electrically charged particles. Any therapy that can positively affect the movement and reactions of molecules within the body can create huge changes in health. I studied polarity therapy in 1980, and I thought it was a helpful therapy because it can balance the body's electrical field. A practitioner can do amazing things with polarity, such as correcting short legs, pulling stress out of the system, as well as helping various types of physiological dysfunctions. In addition, polarity therapy can improve overall health.

Therapeutic touch was discovered and developed by nurses practicing in hospitals and rehabilitation centers. In therapeutic touch, practitioners move their hands over the body's energy field in a certain pattern. When the energetic field of the patient is balanced by using therapeutic touch, practitioners have noted that patients' health generally seemed to improve, and they usually had decreased recovery time.

Magnets

Magnets have been used for centuries to aid the healing process. This old form of healing was reinvented in the 1980s by several companies that designed magnets primarily for pain reduction. Many other therapeutic benefits have been rediscovered with this resurgence. This includes decreased injury recovery time, improved energy, enhanced sleep and better overall health.

How energy medicine works

In China, acupuncture, tai chi and qi gong are ways of energizing, strengthening, reducing stress and balancing the body in order to assist the healing process of any condition, including preventing future illness. These therapies all make extensive use of the energetic systems of the body. These are medically proven protocols in China that have been in place for thousands of years. However, most Americans know little of their benefits.

Many types of electromagnetic energy fields exist in our world today. These include gravitational fields, light beams, sound waves, geopathic energy, cell and cordless phone frequencies, radio and television airwaves, electromagnetic energy from appliances, televisions and computers, and etheric energy, such as auras. Many of these energies are chaotic in nature, and it is unpredictable how the body's balanced internal environment has to deal with this constant bombardment and negative accumulation. These negative energies are called electromagnetic smog, and they are much more prevalent in large cities.

Notice how your body feels after just a short time on the cell phone or in front of your computer. Many people feel a bit off and slightly more tense. This is due to the altered biochemical reactions that cause electromagnetic disturbances within the body. Many people are not aware of their body in this realm of existence. Only time will tell what the effects of these cumulative electromagnetic fields will have on health. Many people find solace in the country or by the ocean where the fields of energetic chaos are much less pronounced.

Every living thing has a live, biomagnetic field around it. Every event, or reaction in the body, produces an electrical charge. The body's own electromagnetic field is greatly influenced by the biomagnetic fields that surround them. The body is constantly taking in this subtle information from the external environment. Molecules within the body feel these disturbances on a cellular level. Each molecule has its own sensors, just like a rabbit sitting with its ears up quietly on alert for the slightest sound. Cells on one end of the body respond to stimulus at the opposite end as each molecule is both sending and receiving information simultaneously, much like an instantaneous transmission of radio frequencies; everyone is getting the exact message at the same time.

Once a resonating molecule receives this signal, it acts on it, or sends a concurrent vibrational signal as a response, so that other molecules can respond in appropriate ways. The cell structures within the cytoplasma (fluid within a cell) are much like musical instruments. Molecules and atoms literally vibrate during this communication process. They carry these messages like harmonic waves from cell to cell within this living matrix. Cell membranes house sensory apparatus components that are able to receive the input and transfer it into the cell. Water is the medium that houses these cell structures and molecules. These molecules are constantly interacting with each other in this water medium. This creates electrical energy throughout the body.

Acupuncture points serve as circuits within each meridian. They operate as input or stimulation centers. These points also function as conductors for electrical information along a pathway called a meridian. Meridians are the main transmission lines, which interconnect with charkas, tissues and cells, right down to the DNA of each cell. Each part of the cell is constantly sending vibratory messages about its current status in relationship to the whole system. When you apply pressure or insert a needle into an acupuncture point, there is a change in polarity, movement of charged ions and shifts in electrical current. That is why with acupuncture treatments you can stimulate a point and have a reaction at the other end of the meridian. This input can then be carried to other areas within that meridian, as well as its paired meridian. The tissues and organs that the meridians transverse become the recipients of this healing energy current (Oschman, 2000).

Collagen fibers are the basic composition of much of the soft tissue such as the muscles, ligaments and tendons. Within these collagen fibers are hollow tubes that are filled with water, according to Mae-Wan Ho, Ph.D. Electrons pass through these tubes. Qi is the movement of electrons within this column of water. These columns of collagen fibers are wrapped in a triple helix configuration. Meridians have a relationship to the structured water columns associated with collagen fibers. Gilbert Ling, Ph.D., has many enlightened concepts that differ some from traditional thinkers in this field as well. He has written several books on cell function and membrane physiology. His understanding goes beyond traditional thinkers in his area of expertise (Ling, 2001).

These two researchers are ahead of their time. For instance, if you were to stimulate spleen six, an acupuncture point on the inside of the ankle, a stimulus of qi would then be directed up the spleen meridian, and into the spleen itself. This is like hooking a jump starter to the spleen. This would strengthen the spleen, as well as any blockages that may be lying along the way. Because the knee and groin are on its path, any problems in the knee or groin area may improve due to the opening up of this energy called qi that runs through these areas. Acupuncture meridians are pathways for electrical flow. Acupuncture seems to balance these circuits, and electrical flow, which is why it can be so effective.

This is another reason the allopathic model of isolating body parts and systems into disease concepts has little understanding of how stressing one organ or body system has to have a rebound effect with another part of the body in another location. The subtle balances of interactions between systems are thrown out of kilter. In allopathic medicine, this always requires the need for more drugs to deal with the compensations that the body constantly has to readjust to. Electromagnetic pathways are choked off from receiving this vital circulating qi. Drugs and surgeries then alter the electromagnetic current within the body. When you cut across or along a meridian in surgery, there is a permanent negative change of electrical conductivity within that meridian. That energetic pathway had been disrupted. Energetic flow is reduced in whatever area and/or organ in which that meridian transverses.

Many people involved either as a patient or a practitioner in alternative health and energy medicine know these types of therapies have great value in a clinical setting. However, the scientific world is generally skeptical about the data behind them. Without this, it has little value to them in terms of its potential for further study or clinical use. Most of the people who are the greatest skeptics of these therapies have never received them, nor have done any research on them. I call these people armchair health experts. That is like only eating one type of food your whole life. You only have knowledge of that food.

Medical science has recently developed various machines that mimic the electrical flow produced by human touch. When humans touch someone as in therapeutic touch, the practitioner's hands give off magnetic currents that oscillate at various frequencies. These are called oscillating magnetic fields. These ranges of frequencies interact with the patient's electromagnetic field. This interaction proceeds to kick start the immune system and other healing mechanisms that greatly need a boost. This inherent touch can be the difference in how effective one's healing process can be. Medical devices are currently being researched and used that produce similar magnetic fields, which are able to penetrate deep into tissues, and have the ability to speed up the healing process of bones, skin and soft tissue. These oscillating currents mimic the exact currents a practitioner of therapeutic touch is able to transfer into a patient's body.

Acupuncture is probably one of the most effective forms of energy healing in its ability to speed up the healing process. Acupuncture and massage are being used more and more in professional settings, including the professional athletic arena. This is due to their ability to not only reduce pain, but to speed up the healing process as well. Every rehabilitation center should have an acupuncturist and massage therapist on staff. Most patients would be able to decrease their time in rehabilitation and heal much more deeply and effectively (Oschman, 2000).

Many of the energy techniques that have been mentioned can cause a change in electrical conductivity, thereby causing shifts in the therapeutic healing process. However, there may be a condition that is an inherent problem within the system, which is much more deeply ingrained than these types of therapies can address. You then have to access much deeper avenues of healing modalities that can make permanent shifts in how the body functions (Oschman, 2000).

Because of the current status of our environment, substances are entering our bodies that are not natural. The ability to work energetically at a cellular level with underlying causative agents, such as lingering pathogens and toxins, and their subsequent reactions, can help shift the healing process to a more permanent basis. This must be accomplished with therapies that can repattern the system energetically or through selective detoxification protocols, so that these corrections can have lasting effects. This is much different from therapy that focuses on moving energy around the body. The patient may feel better temporarily, but the underlying problem is still present. This causative agent will eventually override the system once the treatment wears off. That is why it is so important to differentiate among the various types of energy work, as some can have only temporary results in certain situations. For example, you a have lingering elbow pain that does not seem to get better, no matter what type of therapy you have undertaken. You have tried massage, acupuncture, physical therapy, polarity and Reiki with little results. All seemed to have helped temporarily, but the pain always returned. This is because the treatments you received shifted the effect, but still left the underlying cause. This is not to say that these therapies are not effective in the context in which they were designed. Sometimes blockages can arise that are non-pathogenic, or not related to heavy metals or other toxins. It could be an old injury that never fully healed, which is creating an energetic blockage in your arm.

These scenarios can be great candidates for energy medicine therapies. Removing the blockages either physical or emotional is what is needed to allow the body's innate healing response to kick in. This is like a beaver damming up a river upstream. All you are getting is a trickle of water by the time it reaches you. This is what happens to the energy in your body when it gets to a blockage; major problems arise. I have witnessed many people permanently heal lingering pain problems with acupuncture, massage, polarity therapy, chiropractic or emotional release therapies, because energy blocks were eliminated. By unblocking the river upstream, new healing energy can flow unhindered into areas for healing. Free flowing energy throughout the system is a major key to health.

Energy medicine references

Some excellent books are available on energy medicine. One called *Energy Medicine: The Scientific Basis* by James L. Oschman, Ph.D., shows conclusively the significant science behind these therapies. This book links science and energetic phenomena, revealing how the transference of subtle energy to another human can help stimulate the healing processes.

Notes

Ling, Gilbert, Ph.D. *Life at the Cell and Below-Cell Level: The Hidden History of a Fundamental Revolution in Biology.* Melville, New York, 2001.

Oschman, James L., Ph.D. *Energy Medicine: The Scientific Basis.* London: Churchill Livingstone, 2000.

References

Cecchini, Marie A., M.S., David E. Root, M.D., M.P.H., Jeremie R. Rachunow, M.D., and Phyllis Gelb, M.D. "Chemical Exposures at the World Trade Center," *Townsend Letter for Doctors and Patients*, April 2006.

Deadman, Peter and Mazin Al-Khafaji. *A Manual of Acupuncture.* Vista, California: Eastland Press, 1998.

Lipton, Bruce, Ph.D. "The Wisdom of Your Cells," *Light of Consciousness*, Spring 2007.

Chapter 3: My Story

My healing journey began in my teenage years. I grew up in a hostile environment in Southern California. Survival was the name of the game. When I turned sixteen, I became very ill with severe, non-stop jaw pain that took over my life. I dropped out of high school at seventeen and went from doctor to doctor seeking relief to get healed from this unexpected illness.

Traditional medicine treatments

Medical doctors ran a few tests and basically said there was nothing wrong with me. I would just have to live with the pain. I was distraught from the constant, horrible pain, and was disappointed with the medical system. The stress of trying to attend high school and the pain were unbearable. I started breaking out with acne, so I went to a dermatologist. He prescribed tetracycline that did a great job in clearing up my acne. I stayed on this drug for more than two years. The pain continued the next few years without any let up. I dropped out of high school and life, as each day was a struggle to survive. The pain was constant and ranged from an eight to a ten on a scale of one through ten, with ten being excruciating.

A few years later I started to develop other symptoms that were unexpected. Terrible gas, fatigue, brain fog and depression were added to the pain. I went back to the medical system and saw several medical doctors and neurologists who prescribed various antidepressants. They all failed to help my depression.

Finally, I ended up in a top neurologist's office. He prescribed two new antidepressants that put my nervous system into a frenzy. I kept telling him I felt horrible on this medicine, but he insisted I just was not taking enough. Who was I to question the doctor, especially one who came with such high credentials? I did what he said, took the dosage prescribed and felt even worse. I immediately decided to stop taking the drugs. A week after quitting these medications, I still felt awful. I went to a nurse at my college because I could not make it to the other side of the pool without stopping because my heart was pounding. She informed me that my resting heart rate was 90 and my blood pressure was 136 over 96. Three months earlier my last physical showed my resting heart rate to be 68 and my blood pressure was 96 over 64. The drugs had altered my body's chemistry.

These were important lessons in my healing journey as I began to realize that the traditional medical system was not all it was cracked up to be. I was now twenty years old and still had the chronic pain, depression, brain fog, fatigue and terrible gas.

Something was definitely wrong, but I was not about to go back to the medical doctors so they could experiment on me with any more of their toxic drugs.

Alternative medicine treatments

I then met an alternative medical doctor who prescribed large doses of certain vitamins and amino acids to help with the depression. That did not work either, but at least I was not worse off. I kept searching for answers and became interested in natural cures. I decided to see a macrobiotic adviser who could help me with my diet. He had no degree and did not charge much, so I figured, "What the heck?" After telling him my symptoms and history, he said I might have something called *Candida albicans*. I had not heard of this before. He explained that taking antibiotics for such a long period probably caused the candida, which is like a yeast infection in the intestinal tract. He told me to eat only protein and veggies for a few days and see how I felt. By the third day my depression and spaciness had improved significantly and so did my fatigue and gas problem. I began researching candida and developed an understanding about how my symptoms were related to taking the antibiotics years earlier. I still had the horrible jaw pain, but as long as I stayed on this diet, the post-antibiotic symptoms were nonexistent. I had gone to all of these trusted health experts, and not only did they not have a clue as to what was causing my pain, but they added several new problems with their drugs. The person who helped me the most had no formal degree or license. He knew more than the "medical" experts about my problems. I was on a search for natural methods, but had no idea how long or which direction this journey would lead. What I learned most of all was to trust myself and not assume that a proper degree or following what everyone else was doing was the right thing for me.

My first experience with an alternative practitioner was a man named Lawrence Crusoe. He was an ex-chiropractor in his eighties who worked out of the basement of his home. He did not adjust me like a chiropractor, but did polarity therapy in conjunction with nutritional education. I would spend an hour with him for a grand total of ten dollars. He was my first teacher in a long list to come. This was in the early 1980s.

During this time my wife developed lymph cancer called Hodgkin's disease. She went through traditional chemotherapy, but the cancer returned within a year. She then went to Stanislav Burzynski, M.D., in Houston, Texas, who worked with supporting the immune system instead of tearing it down as chemotherapy does. Within a few months the cancer was totally gone and to this day she is alive and healthy. This was another big lesson along my journey.

The 1980s were filled with learning, some good and some not so good, as lessons can take many forms. Emotional work was being incorporated into my healing process as I learned how this could have a powerful effect on healing and happiness, as well as my jaw pain. I was slowly getting better; however, it was not fast enough for me. I was now incorporating more mega supplements into my plan.

In 1984, I received my massage license so I could practice holistic health. My jaw pain was still a huge factor, as it limited my ability to be myself and function effectively, though it had improved some, mainly due to the emotional work and my restricted diet. I lost more than seventy pounds during this time and weighed 130 pounds. My energy was good as long as I stayed on the candida diet. As soon as I went off the diet, I would start to feel worse again. For all these years, I was in survival mode, but never gave up hope in my search for answers.

In the late 1980s, I met a certified Touch for Health instructor who practiced applied kinesiology (muscle testing). This really interested me as I was looking for other treatment modalities besides bodywork. With muscle testing, I could test myself and my patients for food and vitamin sensitivities. I could determine if people were sensitive to certain foods and/or their vitamins. They could then avoid them once identified. This was just the beginning of what my future focus was to become.

Alternative medicine training

In 1990, I took a Contact Reflex Analysis course. This technique uses muscle testing and acupuncture points to determine the overall functioning of the person. It was exciting work as we could pinpoint for the first-time weaknesses, deficiencies and blockages within the system and use specific nutritional products to balance these. It seemed like a unique and precise method to incorporate into my practice.

I was also learning from other healers and lecturers the importance of detoxification. This meant cleaning out the internal body, specifically the liver, kidneys, colon and lymph system. Using herbal cleansers for this purpose seemed to help some people feel better and become healthier.

As the 1990s progressed, I became more interested in working with internal disorders and knew that my days as a body worker were coming to an end. I, however, was realizing that the scope of contact reflex analysis could only go so far. I did not feel that much better despite taking more than three hundred dollars worth of supplements per month. The jaw pain was slightly better as I discovered that I had a nightshade food sensitivity that was causing increased pain. I was abstaining from eating these foods and continued on the candida diet. I also tried all types of antifungal and probiotics (live microbial feed supplements) to get rid of the horrible candida problem. However, despite my hard work, I still had a good case of candida, as I could not shake it. I was becoming a bit disillusioned with alternative methods as my health hit a standstill. I was tired of such restrictions in my lifestyle and hoped someone had a better approach.

In 1994, my practice was more focused on applied kinesiology. One of my patient's sister was a medical doctor in Alaska. She told me about a new bioenergetic technique that was permanently ridding people of their allergic sensitivities. Her sister was having good success with this method. Since Connie (my client) suffered from many sensitivities, she urged me to travel to California for training. I was not interested in working with sensitivities, but was more interested in getting rid of this dreaded candida, both for my patients and myself. I called the creator of this technique and asked her about her success in treating candida. She replied that her allergy technique could help get my candida under control, but she could not explain how this worked physiologically. I hung up thinking she was just another person promising results without any concrete explanation. I told Connie I really did not have the funds for the training and that I was not interested in working with people who had sensitivities. She handed me a check for half the class tuition and urged me again to take it. I explained this to my next client whose son had allergies, and she handed me a check for the other half of the tuition. They both agreed that I could repay them by practicing this technique with them after I completed the training.

Someone above was telling me something, so I decided to listen. I signed up for the next class and flew to Los Angeles for the first training. I remember sitting down in the class and seeing a huge sign up front that said, "Allergies are everything." I laughed to myself and thought, "No way." I took the training, but was skeptical of the work.

Months went by and the sensitivity kit from the class that I had purchased, along with the workbook, stayed in my drawer. I had taken the class in February of 1994, and it was now late June. Cathy, who had given me half the class money, was fighting a severe bronchial cold. She was very sick and the supplements she was taking to fight it off were not working. She was desperate and said that she was going to get some antibiotics the next day if I could not help her. I remembered that the allergy work had a way in which I could support her immune system's response to the infectious agents that were causing her symptoms, similar to an allergy. I then supported her immune system's response to the lingering pathogens that were invading her lungs. She called me the next day and said her symptoms had improved dramatically following the treatment and that she had not needed the antibiotics after all. I did not understand how it could have worked, but thought maybe there was something to this work. The following week my son became sick, after moving into a new mobile home. His allergies had become much worse. I cleared him for three sensitivities including vitamin C. We were both surprised he felt a lot better.

Now it was time to use myself as a guinea pig. I never thought I was an allergic person, besides an occasional shellfish reaction. I did not sneeze or have any typical allergy symptoms, but I began testing myself for sensitivities. I was startled to find that I tested weak for many of the nutrients that I was taking. Several of the vitamin B complexes were weak, as was calcium and others, including many sugars. These are some of the basic ten nutritional sensitivities that are the starting point for the treatment protocol. My first treatment was on some of the B vitamins. Within a few days following the treatment, I remember feeling somewhat better. I had a bit more energy and felt calmer. This was interesting, because that is exactly what B complex is supposed to do. I was taking mega doses of B vitamins prior to this, but never before felt this effect. Could I have been sensitive to B complex all of my life and just needed it reprogrammed into my body so they would be compatible with my system? During the next three months, I treated myself every day as I found new sensitivities to numerous substances that I did not know one could be sensitive to. I remember that a few years earlier I took a handful of minerals that came from the Great Salt Lake. They were high in electrolytes and salt. I was so spacy from taking them that I ran my car into my garage. When I cleared my salt sensitivity, I could feel a substantial amount of mental fog subside. I then realized that salt was in almost everything I ate, as it was a sensitivity that I did not react to immediately, but was a chronic symptomatic reaction that was always there. I thought my mental fog was part of how my brain functioned, not knowing that it was my sensitivity to salt that was behind the brain fog. I went on to clear all of the basic nutrients and was finally starting to feel good. Clearing magnesium made a huge shift in the way I felt. My muscles started to relax for the first time in my life and I felt instantly calmer. I had been taking huge amounts of magnesium prior to this for that reason, but never before felt this effect.

I attended the second allergy training as I gained more confidence with the method. I also started to test my brain chemicals for sensitivities. I found I was sensitive to several of these chemicals including serotonin, epinephrine as well as tryptophan, an amino acid that helps produce serotonin. The most amazing treatment I had was for serotonin. Immediately upon finishing the treatment, I felt like the last cloud was lifted out of my brain. I could think better as my mind was suddenly clear. It was amazing to feel so different with one treatment, like someone had turned on a light switch that had been in the off position all my life. I next cleared myself for candida. It took ten days to complete the treatment and the diet. Once done, I started to eat foods I had not eaten for years. Fruit, cake, cookies and, yes, ice cream without any reactions at all. I could not believe that this amazing technique had given me my life back. I had so much energy that I remember staying up every night until two o'clock in the morning reading. I also put on thirty pounds during the next three months as I ate everything in sight. I was forty years old now and my life was just beginning.

I decided to attend acupuncture school. I moved to Seattle and started my sensitivity repatterning practice. Within a few months my practice took off. I was attending school full time, and had a full-time practice. Twelve-hour days were the norm including weekends. I had put my life on hold for so long, and, finally, I was doing what I wanted in life. I was out of the survival mode forever. I continued my practice until I finished school. Completely exhausted, I took a long break and then decided to practice in Arizona.

One day a client showed me an article in *Alternative Medicine* magazine that looked somewhat like the allergy repatterning technique that I practiced. However, the focus was on pathogens (microscopic "bugs") that were triggering autoimmune diseases and other symptoms. The allergy repatterning was great for sensitivities, but did not focus much on pathogens. I had an instructor in acupuncture school who talked in-depth about how lingering pathogens were causing so much illness. But she said that Traditional Chinese Medicine did not have a very effective treatment method for lingering pathogens. This stuck in my mind as some people like me who received the allergy response repatterning treatments got better. However, others did not seem to improve much, or very little. I knew something was missing. Could this be it?

I was on a plane for the first workshop within weeks. I took several of these trainings, as they were progressive in the material that was presented. I started to work with many seriously ill patients who had a host of autoimmune, as well as other serious disorders. They came in droves with conditions diagnosed by allopathic medicine as arthritis, colitis, fibromyalgia and many others. The basic premise of this work was that lingering pathogens were causing the immune system to attack the body, which made total sense to me and most of my patients. The body is very smart and does things in accordance with certain laws. Naturally, if there was a bug in a certain part of the body, the immune system would attack it, because that is its job. The problem is that the immune system fails to get it out, but keeps trying. The inflammation then is an effect of these ongoing attacks.

Since that time my success rate with chronic conditions has greatly improved in conjunction with my ability to understand the root causes behind the symptoms. I believe my path in life took some rough roads so that I could be motivated enough to search endlessly for the answers to not only my health issues, but the ones that were presenting themselves in my office on a daily basis. I have been able to help thousands of people over the years because of my dedication, knowledge and clinical experience. I am in my sixties now and my health has improved significantly. I believe that what is contained in *An Integrative Approach to Healing Chronic Illness: Revealing the Root Causes of Modern Disease* is the truth, which can only help others find their way back to wholeness again.

References

Cutler, Ellen W., D.C. *Winning the War Against Asthma and Allergies: A Drug-Free Cure for Asthma and Allergy Suffers*. Albany, New York: Delmar Publishers, 1998.

Deadman, Peter and Mazin Al-Khafaji. *A Manual of Acupuncture*. Vista, California: Eastland Press, 1998.

Leviton, Richard. "Say Goodbye to Allergies," *Alternative Medicine*, May 1999.

Chapter 4: The Big Picture

When a patient comes into my office for the first time, I spend an hour with him to establish a basis for the big picture; how we are going to put the pieces back together to achieve health. It can be complicated as the layers may be very deep.

A huge puzzle

The way I see a patient's ailments resembles a huge puzzle that needs to be initially unraveled and then put back together over time. I cannot count the times a patient has come into my practice with layers upon layers of pathogens, sensitivities, toxins and organs that are functioning at a low level. I explain that it will be a slow process and they need to be patient the first month or so because the foundation of their "house" is where we need to start rebuilding. Why fix the cracks in the walls if the foundation is on shaky ground? We must start there, which may not translate immediately into relief of their symptoms. Patients have a huge bag of boulders and rocks that they are dragging around. Taking out a rock or two and a boulder may not change their overall symptoms initially because there are still twenty or so rocks, boulders and even some pebbles that they are still carrying. However, if we can repeat the removal process, fairly soon the bag will become lighter as more rocks and boulders are removed. As more of these obstacles are cleared, they can actually pick up the bag and carry it. Down the road they will be able to run with it. At some point, all the rocks, boulders and even the pebbles will be removed, and the bag can be tossed aside. Healing chronic illness takes time and persistence. Any other way would be a quick patch job that would come apart quickly at the seams.

Underlying or root problems

We have been trained in this country to associate symptoms with illness. We are also trained to believe that suppressing the symptoms is what our goal should be. This mentality has little to do with becoming healthy. The truth is that this way of seeing illness not only fails to address the underlying or root problem, but also allows these deep issues to continue to fester and develop underneath "the blanket" of suppressed symptoms. We have been sold a bill of goods that says, "Take this wonder pill and all of your problems will be better." This also applies to some natural supplements that claim to be the total answer. I have not found that magical pill in any form. We all want the quick fix, which can be frustrating for those practitioners whose focus is on working on the root cause. Patients have been conditioned to see the quick fix as the baseline for determining if a treatment method will work. This may be true in less complicated matters. However, it is rare to see a small puzzle when you have multiple chronic symptoms. Sometimes I work with these patients and if they are not feeling a lot better by week three, they have one foot out the door. The hardest part is always the beginning, as you must remove blockage after blockage. This is a key time for the patient as sensitivity repatterning and pathogenic clearing is a methodical process. Through this process the internal stress load is gradually reduced on the key organs, as they need time for repair and recovery. It may take up to six months for an organ to completely recover from years of internal abuse. Supplements and glandular extractions may help with this rebuilding process. However, giving a patient herbs, glandular extractions and supplements to heal an organ problem can be shortsighted thinking unless you remove the reason why the organ is being degraded in the first place. This is like having a hole in the bottom of your sink. You keep adding water, but the sink keeps leaking. You have to fix the hole. That is what treating the root cause is all about. Then the supplements can be extremely effective in repairing and healing the body.

Pathogens, sensitivities and toxins are not the whole picture for some patients, as other problems can also cause disruption of health. Glandular problems such as the thyroid, adrenal and glucose utilization problems from a weak pancreas as well as hormone imbalances can create much internal havoc. These issues, many times though, are influenced by the pathogens, as they can enter glands thereby causing deterioration of glandular function. Many thyroid conditions are due to pathogenic invasion of this gland, which can produce either hyper- or hypo-function. That is what usually causes an autoimmune thyroid. Sensitivities that create nutrient deficiencies can weaken glands as well. Suppose you were sensitive to iodine, which causes an iodine deficiency. The thyroid needs iodine for proper functioning just as the blood needs iron so it is not anemic. Glands need proper nourishment like the rest of the body. Heavy metals and toxins can also leach into glands causing dysfunction.

The bottom line is to be patient and look at the improvements even if they are small at first. You might experience a bit more energy during the day and may feel a bit clearer mentally. Eventually the good moments will turn into good days, the good days into good months and soon the illness will be a thing of the past.

References

Abramson, John, M.D. *Overdosed America: The Broken Promise of American Medicine*. New York: Harper Perennial, 2005.

Deadman, Peter and Mazin Al-Khafaji. *A Manual of Acupuncture*. Vista, California: Eastland Press, 1998.

Garritano, Joanna, M.D. "U.S. Health Care Puts Profit Over People," *Seattle Post-Intelligencer*, January 10, 2007.

Moynihan, Ray and Alan Cassels. *Selling Sickness: How the World's Biggest Pharmaceutical Companies Are Turning Us All Into Patients*. New York: Nation Books, 2005.

Oschman, James L., Ph.D. *Energy Medicine: The Scientific Basis*. London: Churchill Livingstone, 2000.

Chapter 5: The Disease Process

Many times a patient comes to into my office and asks me how he developed such a horrible illness. Most patients are looking for the one thing that turned their health sour. Most want the one thing that will turn it around. Many have been to all types of health experts, looking for the magic drug or herbal concoction that will turn the tide. My answer is almost always the same. Illness is a process. You did not get this way overnight and probably will not get rid of it that quickly. Quick remedies only exist in movies, fairy tales and drug commercials. Many of my patients have chronic illnesses. It is challenging, but can also be rewarding when they gradually regain their health and get life back.

Here are some ideas about how chronic illnesses occur.

The birth process and early years

Hopefully, a newborn baby named Jimmy was lucky enough to avoid a forceps delivery, which can cause permanent cranial damage. Also, it would be fortunate if Jimmy's mom was not given drugs before and during the birth process. If she was, those drugs were given to Jimmy. How many stories have we heard of drugs causing birth defects or other complications later on?

For this example, we will say Jimmy had an excellent delivery without complications. At six months old, he gets an earache, and his mom, being a good responsible parent, takes him to her favorite pediatrician who prescribes antibiotics. Jimmy feels better because the antibiotics reduced whatever bacteria were in his eustachian tube. Everyone is relieved as the crying subsides. Then a few months later his earache returns, and the same process takes place. Off to the doctor Jimmy goes, and another round of antibiotics is given. The pain subsides and everyone is happy again. Then a few months later Jimmy has a rash that will not go away. He seems to be catching more and more colds. That earache is back again. The third round of antibiotics is prescribed and the symptoms subside once again. Jimmy starts to develop a stuffy nose, which his mom thinks might be an allergy, but it does not go away. One day Jimmy has a full-blown sinus infection. Back to the doctor he goes and guess what he gets for that sinus infection? Another round of antibiotics.

During his early years, Jimmy received more than twenty vaccinations in order to prevent various dreaded diseases. His mom and dad have been good, responsible parents doing what they and their doctor think are best for his health. Jimmy has been to only top physicians since birth. The only problem is that he does not feel well and keeps getting sick. The doctor visits become a common occurrence.

What has actually occurred so far? A child like Jimmy probably was either born with or acquired a bacterial infection from mom in the hospital or at home during the early months. *Staphylococcus aureus*, which causes staph infection, is the most common bacterium that hospitals and society in general have to deal with today. Its favorite hiding places are the ears and sinus cavities. Because a child's eustachian tubes have not yet developed, they have a tendency to be a great host site for bacteria. The antibiotic knocked it down which relieved the pain, but did not kill it. The bug survived it, mutated and is still present in the ear. As time goes on this bacterium starts to grow again and causes the second ear infection. It survives round two of antibiotic warfare. However, this time it mutates to a stronger form. It starts to flourish again and guess where it ventures to? The sinus cavities become its next vacation destination. These cavities are in close proximity to the eustachian tubes. Just a bus transfer away, and they are making a new home in the big city, the sinus cavities. Here come the antibiotics to address the sinus infection, which it again is able to knock down. But the sinus infections keep coming back because the bug was never removed.

Now the child is eight years old and has been on antibiotics at least ten times. Jimmy seems to catch cold after cold and now seems to get diarrhea intermittently. He has bags under the eyes and complains frequently about not feeling well and seems tired a lot. The next trip is to the allergist who performs the famous skin prick tests and determines there is a mold and corn allergy. After repeated series of shots, nothing seems to change.

The teenage years

Jimmy is now in the teenage years, a stressful time as his hormones kick in. His acne is getting worse, so he goes to the dermatologist. Guess what the miracle medicine is that will put a halt to that dreaded acne? You guessed it, another antibiotic called tetracycline. This time, instead of the normal ten-day protocol, the doctor prescribes it for a minimum of one month or until his face clears up. The acne starts to abate and Jimmy starts to look like his old pre-acne self. However, he still does not feel all that well. Jimmy is still getting sick quite often and has a constant low-grade sinus infection that never seems to go away. His nose is always running and/or stuffy, so he takes an over-the-counter medicine that helps temporarily. While on the antibiotics, Jimmy experiences several severe bouts of diarrhea and seems to be a bit more irritable and depressed. He has a hard time focusing on his schoolwork. Jimmy does not have the energy he once did when he was younger. Jimmy goes back to the doctor again to explain his dilemma, because he does not understand what is happening. The doctor thinks that maybe Ritalin might be the answer to help the focus problem, but admits that he does not know why Jimmy is having other symptoms. "Maybe it is the pressure of teenage years and high school," he says. This sounds very possible, so Jimmy thanks him for his insightful diagnosis. Jimmy starts on the Ritalin and within a few days he notices that his focus has improved and he thinks the drug is working well.

The twenties

By the time Jimmy reaches his late twenties, he has been on antibiotics more than twenty times and has a constant gamut of chronic symptoms that will not go away. Jimmy now has a lot of gas, which is embarrassing at times. He also notices that his digestion seems a bit sluggish. The diarrhea is more regular, so his doctor puts him on a stool hardener. Jimmy quit taking the Ritalin because of the side effects and is now taking Prozac, because his depression and inability to focus are getting worse. His doctor is now recommending sinus surgery to clean out his chronically infected sinus cavities. Jimmy drinks three or four cups of coffee a day to have enough energy to get through the day. He hardly exercises anymore because he is too tired after work. Jimmy's girlfriend wonders why he is not feeling well.

The forties

At forty years old, Jimmy has had two failed sinus surgeries. He takes blood pressure medicine and a statin drug to help bring his blood pressure and cholesterol down because it is out of the range of the newly revised guidelines. Jimmy is still taking antibiotics routinely for colds and sinus infections. He has switched to a different antidepressant because he could no longer tolerate the side effects of Prozac. Jimmy has no libido, so at the request of his wife he is taking Viagra in order to perform. His heartburn is getting pretty bad, so his doctor recommended that he change from taking an antacid to a wonderfully colored pill, which he must take daily. The doctor thinks Jimmy may have gastric reflux disease. Jimmy gets reoccurring headaches, so the doctor prescribes a strong pain killer for those severe headaches, which he takes in addition to over-the-counter painkillers.

By his late forties, Jimmy is taking over twenty pills a day. He no longer has a gallbladder as the doctors removed it a few years ago during exploratory surgery. The doctors could not figure out why Jimmy's digestion and elimination were so bad. They said his gallbladder looked diseased when they went in. Following surgery, Jimmy got a staph infection in the hospital that kept him there for ten days. He was on intravenous antibiotic therapy for this infection. Jimmy's energy level is so low that his doctor mentions that he may have something called chronic fatigue syndrome and possibly fibromyalgia, as he seems to have a lot of muscle pain and soreness.

One day at work Jimmy's business partner coughed all over the office. Within a few days Jimmy had the same bug, but his coughing never quit. Jimmy is still coughing three months later. He needs to take more time off from work, as he is tired and constantly getting sick. Whenever someone in the office comes in with a cold, Jimmy seems to get it. He has seen a slow degradation in his health since he was very young. Jimmy does not understand it, because he has been consistent with his doctor visits and done exactly what he was told without questioning. Jimmy has been a good patient and always followed doctor's orders. The funny thing is that even his doctor does not know why he feels the way he does. Jimmy has been to the best doctors and specialists possible, but no one has answers. All they can do is prescribe a drug to help with his symptoms. Jimmy hopes they can figure out what is wrong with him soon, or he may have to quit his job. Jimmy has a friend who swears by his alternative medicine doctor. Jimmy does not believe in that stuff. If modern medicine cannot help him, how could something that is unproven in the scientific world? Alternative medicine is not science-based medicine. Besides if there were a cure for him, surely his doctor would know.

A common story

Jimmy's sad story unfortunately is a common one in society today. Many of our Baby Boom generation have been through a somewhat similar journey. There might be some variances, but the general theme is much the same. A slow degradation of health occurs, as people trust in what they were taught to believe in: drugs, surgery and modern medicine. Had Jimmy received another perspective on his health problems from different types of doctors or practitioners, perhaps he would have changed his path and quite possibly been on his way back to health. Some people have a preconceived notion about alternative medicine that puts up a wall or mental block. They will stick with what does not work, no matter how bad their health deteriorates. Their belief is in an illusion enforced over and over again by traditional medicine and the medical media. This illusion can block them from examining healthier options that might actually be able to treat the root cause of their illness. Jimmy did not do any research on his own. He only consulted with traditional medical doctors who tend to see things through a one-color lens. He refused help from a friend who had discovered for himself that alternative medicine did work.

It is amazing to me to see people in this plight. You want to help them, but they refuse your help because of their rigid belief system. They do not see the value in investing in their health with natural methods. However, they spend a small fortune on co-pays for their numerous prescriptions in the never-ending game of chasing symptoms around the body. They have racked up a history of surgeries, drugs, office visits and countless tests costing thousands upon thousands of dollars. They feel horrible and know their health is deteriorating, but they will continue to go down that straight and narrow path until the end. They are in a tunnel that gets darker and darker the further they venture. They bought the media programming, hook, line and sinker. They never once stopped to assess the methodology, because they have been well schooled to not question medical science. We can go back and see early on how the antibiotics and symptom-oriented medicine created Jimmy's downward spiral. The sad thing is that this is not a fairy tale, but the reality of how our modern health care system operates. Drugs and surgery have little in common with treating the root cause of illness. They actually contribute to keeping you sick by practicing "disease management."

References

Abramson, John, M.D. *Overdosed America: The Broken Promise of American Medicine*. New York: Harper Perennial, 2005.

Garritano, Joanna, M.D. "U.S. Health Care Puts Profit Over People," *Seattle Post-Intelligencer*, January 10, 2007.

Snyder Sachs, Jessica. "Are Antibiotics Killing Us?" *Discover*, November 2005.

"'Watch and Wait'–A Shift in Approach to Kids' Ear Infections," Pediatrics/Children's Health News, June 6, 2005.

Chapter 6: The Healing Process

Every patient that comes into my office wants to be healed yesterday. Many are in a survival mode when they first come in; every day is a challenge just to get through it. Many cannot function at a job. They do not understand how many things are compromising their health. Some want that magic pill for their numerous symptoms and are reluctant to spend the time and money it takes to get well. They want me to figure out the one thing that is causing all of this. In all my years of treating chronic patients, I cannot remember when it was one thing, or even two things. Problems are usually layered. What do I mean by the term layered? They have a large puzzle to be put back together. They are dragging a large bag behind, loaded with rocks and boulders. They did not get sick overnight. There were many factors that brought them to their present condition. It is only logical thinking that healing will return gradually because they did not become ill overnight.

A difficult puzzle

Have you ever put together a large difficult puzzle? At first you look at it and say, "I have no clue where anything goes." However, after you figure out one section and put that together then a few other sections, soon the whole picture starts to reveal itself. Healing chronic illness is much the same. You may fix a couple of the major pieces and some of the symptoms may improve or even disappear. You will still have other variables that may still be there, but you can start to see how the rest of the puzzle is laid out. The overall picture gets less and less fuzzy as you clear the debris.

The more allergies, pathogens and toxins patients have directly correlates to how sick they are. This will determine how much work and time it will take to get well. The more drugs and surgeries they have had, the slower the recovery will be. Surgeries cut into the vital acupuncture meridians impeding the energy flow. Drugs are poison to the system.

Once in a while I will have a fairly healthy person come in for some obscure problem. Healthy people usually have few toxins, pathogens and allergies.

As allergies, pathogens and toxins are removed, the puzzle gets smaller and smaller, and the chronically ill patient usually begins to feel much better. Remember, symptoms are just effects. The allergies, nutritional deficiencies (usually from the allergies), pathogens, toxins and subsequent organ degradation create these effects.

The right practitioner

If the problems patients are having are mostly pathogenic, then that is the particular specialty they need to seek out. Choosing a practitioner who specializes in detoxification instead is like trying to nail down a roof with only a saw. Patients will not get much better because the source of their problem did not match the specialty of the practitioner they needed. I have had a few patients tell me that they do not believe alternative medicine works because they received treatments from one healer who happened to specialize in an area other than what they needed, which is absurd. There can be many specialties within a scope of practice that may be the one, or a combination of things that is needed for recovery. People must stay open to seeking relief to suffering and not give up. Research for the right therapy and practitioner is the key. The people that do their own research are the ones who eventually get well.

Sometimes it can take years before all the right pieces are revealed and put back into place. Patience is the key to everything as far as healing is concerned; in the long run persistence will usually pay off in great dividends. Steady process over time certainly beats no progress in a short time.

Health regained

When the pathogens, allergies and toxins are finally cleared out, patients return to a balanced state and can view life from that healthy perspective. They can then look back and see the gradual changes over time. Once patients reach the top of the mountain it is much easier to look down and see all the obstacles that had to be cleared away in order to reach the top. When they are at the bottom looking up without a map, or clear path in front of them, then it is very difficult and confusing, especially when they have been led down several paths that looked promising but resulted in a dead end. When health is regained or found for the first time, many patients tell me that they had forgotten what it was like to be healthy. Some never knew what it felt like because they were sick for so long. A job they thought they would have to quit because they were too sick to work becomes the job they want to leave because they need a bigger challenge. Employees who do not have enough energy to excel at their jobs can regain their power once again.

When patients regain their health, they get their life back and everything changes for the better. Sometimes even relationships will take on a different perspective. Getting well is a process, and if people can look at it in that manner then good things can happen for them. If people are shown a way or means of getting well, which helps them to understand how they got sick in the first place, then they usually are more open and hopeful.

Too many health care practitioners do not really understand the causes of chronic illness. Therefore, when they are challenged by a difficult case, they are guessing at best as to the cause, let alone a cure. Many of these practitioners are good capable people with expertise in their particular specialty. The problem lies with the lack of current information that can expose the source of these chronic illnesses. A practitioner must understand the potential for allergies, lingering pathogens and toxicity, as key causative agents in chronic illness. Otherwise, practitioners may not have the insight and the proper tools to deal with complex illness. This is why so many patients with complicated causes get minimal or no improvement, despite various treatments and thousands of dollars spent on supplements. People need a hammer to nail things down, not a saw. Keep searching until you find the right combination of healers who have the proper tools for what you need. They are out there, so keep looking.

References

Deadman, Peter and Mazin Al-Khafaji. *A Manual of Acupuncture*. Vista, California: Eastland Press, 1998.

Oschman, James L., Ph.D. *Energy Medicine: The Scientific Basis*. London: Churchill Livingstone, 2000.

Chapter 7: Mechanisms of Damage

There is a huge difference in how the body sustains damage between an acute infection and a chronic infection. If you hurt your elbow by falling on it, you will have an inflammatory reaction. However, as long as you take care of it and do not reinjure it, all the inflammation will be gone and things will eventually return to normal. However, if for some reason lingering inflammation continues, then over time the body will start to protect it by laying down scar tissue in the form of collagen or calcium depending upon which type of tissue is under stress. Calcium tends to help with bone protection, while collagen helps with soft tissue. This process helps with repair, but also tends to limit movement in order to protect itself from further damage. White blood cells are usually called to the injury site at first in order to help with the healing and inflammatory process. Macrophages are usually first in line. They stimulate other white blood cells by releasing cytokines and leukotrienes, which are chemicals that attract more white blood cells. They also stimulate other cells to build up and repair damaged tissue.

Chronic infection

When the stimulus is chronic, then lymphocytes become part of the long-term picture. White blood cells are the body's army. Their order is always to seek out and destroy. When this process goes on beyond the acute stage, delicate tissues become damaged. This process can take years, even decades to manifest. The damage slowly takes its toll.

Typically, many of my patients feel fine until their thirties. They would notice feeling aches and pains on and off, but always attributed it to something else. Their energy would slowly decline, which they attributed to getting older. Many times they forgot how they used to feel. At some point, they start to wonder if there was something wrong. By the time they reach their forties, the pain has become chronic, and they have a host of other symptoms that have crept up gradually over the years.

You cannot see a lingering pathogen causing a chronic low-grade infection in your knee joint, or in your brain. However, you can tell when the thinking processes are declining, and you can hardly get up in the morning because your knee is so stiff. You just feel the symptoms, but cannot see or understand the cause.

Damage from chronic infection

Over time, the tissue that is chronically inflamed will eventually sustain some damage. The cartilage is the most vulnerable part of the joint. Chronic joint inflammation leads to degeneration of the cartilage. The heart valves are the most delicate structure of the heart. This is why we see so much heart valve damage. Lung and liver tissue can become fibrotic (abnormal fibrous tissue has developed) after years of inflammation. Lung fibrosis places a burden on the heart because of decreased oxygen utilization. The heart then must work harder to pump the oxygen-rich blood to the arteries. Chronic ear infections cause hearing loss due to damage to the eardrum. Chronic eye infections lead to cornea and lens damage, which causes decreased vision and blindness in some cases. Chronic low-grade brain inflammation leads to headaches, Alzheimer's, bipolar disorder, tumors, depression, schizophrenia, reduced brain function and, yes, brain damage. Long-term inflammation in the bowels causes damage to the mucosal lining of the intestinal tract. This reduces your ability to digest and absorb nutrients. It also leads to leaky gut syndrome. There are very few structures in the body that can stand up to long-term, low-grade inflammation without showing the effects. The muscles are the most resilient. I often joke with patients and say, "If you are going to have an inflammatory disease, it is best to have chronic muscle inflammation because the muscles are difficult to damage."

Remember, it is not the pathogens that do the major damage; it is the response to the pathogens by the immune system that destroys tissue. The bugs are the gun, and the immune system's response, which is producing the chronic inflammation, becomes the bullet. Therefore, damage is always the end result of any prolonged inflammatory condition. Reversing the process goes like this: tissue damage is produced by the inflammation, which follows the cause of the inflammation. Barring physical injury, it is usually lingering pathogens causing the chronic infection. It is that simple.

References

Dvonch, Louis, M.D., and Russell Dvonch. *The Heart Attack Germ: Prevent Strokes, Heart Attacks, and the Symptoms of Alzheimer's by Protecting Yourself From the Infections and Inflammation of Cardiovascular Disease*. New York: Writer's Showcase, 2003.

Nicolson, Garth L, Ph.D. "Chronic Infectious Diseases," The Institute for Molecular Medicine, Accessed June 26, 2005. www.immed.org/illness/fatigue_illness_research.html

Ojcius, David M., Toni Darville and Patrick M. Bavoil. "Can Chlamydia Be Stopped?" *Scientific American*, May 2005.

Chapter 8: Organ Degradation

As we age our bodies naturally and gradually slow down. However, if we take good care of ourselves this process will be very slow. We should all have good energy and organ function well into our nineties. If this is true, why do people begin declining in their forties? It has a lot to do with lifestyle, which includes diet, stress and other factors. The chief organs in Chinese medicine are the liver, kidneys and spleen. These are referred to as the yin organs. As their deterioration escalates, then illness and fatigue will set in.

Chinese medicine theories

Chinese medicine believes that the kidneys are the root organ. They are your batteries and are the basis for sexual and physical energy. If your kidneys are determined to be weak in this ancient medical model, you would be diagnosed as having a kidney qi or kidney yin deficiency problem. You would be given some herbal tonics and acupuncture to boost the kidneys. You may also be counseled on ways in which you are expending too much kidney energy in your life. Overwork, stress and excessive sex for males can wear down your internal batteries, which is your kidney essence.

The role of pathogens, toxins and heavy metals

I want to take you a bit upstream from this perspective. In my reasoning, when I know that a patient has low kidney function, I will always start out by giving him herbs and acupuncture, because it will be most helpful to support the kidneys. However, my overall understanding of why the kidneys are weak differs somewhat from Traditional Chinese Medicine. I am not trying to degrade a three-thousand-year-old method that has proven itself far beyond question. However, I would like to explain it from a different perspective.

In China three thousand years ago, they did not have pollution as we do today. Life was not nearly as stressful. Mercury was not being put into their mouths, nor was it accumulated in the fish they ate. The public was not being vaccinated with the twenty or so vaccines that we are told today that we need. Many of the hybrid pathogens that we deal with today were not lurking back then. Antibiotics were not available, so *Candida albicans* and *Clostridium difficile*, as well as other mutated pathogens, did not exist. Allergies were not really a part of Chinese medicinal philosophy. For that time and culture, the Chinese system of medicine was very effective. It is still very effective for most of the wide range of health issues we are challenged with today. However, we may need to add other complementary modalities and protocols to fully address the root causes of some of the seriously chronic conditions created by the toxins, heavy metals, allergies and lingering pathogens that we must deal with on a daily basis. These are complicated causes, and their makeup is not part of a natural disease process.

Pathogens degrade organs in several ways. First and foremost, any pathogen can take residence in any organ of the body. We have all heard of someone with kidney disease caused by a virus or bacteria that takes over the organ. Secondly, from a purely physiological perspective, the kidneys are filters in the body. This means that they filter waste material. Toxic byproducts of the inflammatory processes created by antigen/antibody complexes are produced and released into the bloodstream when a white blood cell attacks a pathogen. If the attacks are chronic, these byproducts are being released constantly. This creates an acidic cellular environment, which adds to the inflammatory condition, the kidneys must continually filter this all out. The kidneys become run down because they constantly have to dump these toxins. When I feel a patient's kidneys and they feel tired, it is easy to understand why they are in this condition. The kidneys feel like they want to say, "Give me a vacation. I am about to check out." The feeling I get is pure exhaustion. I then know that this patient has probably several lingering pathogens or toxic internal debris that is placing a toll on the kidneys. Nutritional and herbal support and acupuncture specific to the kidneys can definitely be helpful. Often this may only be addressing the effect in this scenario as an organ is run down for a reason. It does not just happen by accident as something, or a combination of things, is pulling it down.

The kidneys

The kidneys are like your batteries. Suppose you had a ten-year battery in your car but worked it four times as hard. How long do you think it would last? That is what takes place with the kidneys. They just get overworked without a break. They are putting in overtime and working weekends. When pathogens are removed from the system and the toxic load is reduced, the kidneys start to come back on their own. They recover even faster with acupuncture, herbal tonics and cleansers. Many chronic patients are in this degradation condition. I use acupuncture and herbs with these patients specifically for the kidneys, as they need all the help they can get. It is like a rocket needing a boost to get off the ground. As the immune system removes the pathogens in conjunction with the organ cleansing protocols that are removing toxins from the system as well as from the kidneys themselves, then the burden on the kidneys is reduced and kidney strength is regained. I can then reduce the herbs and acupuncture as the kidney function is restored. This may take months to accomplish as the person may have several pathogens and other complications pulling them down. I might feel the kidneys again several months later. By then, I can usually feel the difference in their life force compared to before. What is being done here is to go "upstream" and rid the body of what was pulling the kidneys down. Allergies and nutritional deficiencies as well as poor diet can also contribute to kidney degradation.

The liver

The next organ is the powerful liver. This organ in Chinese medicine controls the muscles and the blood. It also influences the mind to some degree. Have you ever heard of an angry alcoholic or a woman with PMS? The liver becomes hot in both of these cases and causes the heat to go to the head, which causes anger, rage and irritability. Many cholesterol drugs that affect the liver can cause muscle problems. Even Western medicine can see the connection between the liver and muscles.

Pathogens can also enter the liver. The liver is a chief detoxifier of the blood, similar to the kidneys. The same process as described in the kidneys can take place in the liver. The difference is that an unhealthy liver can become stagnant or stuck. Blood is pooling instead of flowing. It feels strong when you palpate it, but it also feels stuck or stagnant. The liver is saying loud and clear, "Someone please help me get unstuck, free me." The liver may also be deficient. The two diagnoses in Chinese medicine would be liver qi stagnation and liver yin deficiency. Remove the sources of what is causing the problem, and the liver will revive itself. We all know that hepatitis affects the liver, which can eventually cause damage, but other pathogens can live there as well. The liver needs to be cleansed of its toxins. This is usually done with herbs. Acupuncture can also help get it unstuck and boost its energy. When this is done, along with immune supported pathogen extraction, then the liver will usually come back strong with free-flowing energy.

The spleen

The spleen is the third organ in this group and maybe the most important organ in Chinese medicine. This differs very much from how Western medicine perceives it. The spleen in Chinese medicine, along with the kidneys, helps to transport fluids. The spleen is also vital to digestion of food and turning that food into nourishment. It is weakened by a damp climate and certain foods such as sugar and dairy products. I have never understood how this works physiologically, as my Western education is so different, but I have learned over time that the spleen does in fact do what Chinese medicine theory says it does. My background in anatomy and physiology does not coincide with Chinese medical theory. I have learned much from both medical models and have come to respect Chinese medicine more and more. The spleen in the Western medicine model helps with extra storage of blood and consists of lymph tissue. Therefore, it is part of the lymph system. It also produces white blood cells and helps to cleanse the lymphatic system. Since the spleen produces white blood cells, it is a key organ in the defense of the body.

Guess what happens when you have a host of unwanted critters roaming illegally in your body? The spleen must work overtime just like the kidneys. It will become chronically deficient because it is constantly trying to produce white blood cells to fight off the chronic infections. Also, the lymphatic system is the secondary drainage system after the blood. It helps detoxify the waste products that the blood cannot extract. The spleen helps in this process as well. If there is a constant flow of toxic debris from pathogenic/immune responses and other toxins that cannot be eliminated by other means, then the lymph system and spleen can assist. The spleen weakens due to this burden as well. It is working a separate night job just to keep up with the workload. When I palpate a tired spleen, it feels like it wants to yawn and go back to sleep. It says, "Don't wake me up; I just need some rest." The last reason the spleen becomes tired and weak is due to a pathogenic take over. Bacteria love the spleen. *Staphylococcus* and *Streptococcus* easily enter the lymph system from the neck area, which is loaded with lymph nodes. Have you had a cold and discovered that the nodules on your neck get sore and enlarged? They can easily get infected with *Staphylococcus* and *Streptococcus* as well as other bugs. *Candida albicans* has a hankering for the spleen as well. Any pathogen that is traveling through the lymph system can end up in the spleen. Always remember the general rule, anything can go anywhere anytime.

When an organ gets infected with bugs, it can be sore to the touch and may ache due to the inflammation and infection. The kidneys can sometimes cause back pain. Many patients have told me their organs, including the spleen, liver or intestines, just plain hurt. They ask if this is possible, or if it is just their imagination?

Chief players in organ dysfunction

Pathogens, allergies, heavy metals, toxins and poor nutrition are the chief players in organ dysfunction. You have to go upstream and plug the holes so that the organs can rest and have a chance to recover so proper energy or qi can be restored.

References

Deadman, Peter and Mazin Al-Khafaji. *A Manual of Acupuncture*. Vista, California: Eastland Press, 1998.

Giovanni, Maciocia. *The Practice of Chinese Medicine: The Treatment of Diseases With Acupuncture and Chinese Herbs*. London: Churchill Livingstone, 1994.

Oschman, James L., Ph.D. *Energy Medicine: The Scientific Basis*. London: Churchill Livingstone, 2000.

Chapter 9: Disease Management and Modern Medicine

"Disease management" is fairly new as it reflects how allopathic medicine treats illness in our present time. Disease management simply implies that diseases, which seem to be growing in types and numbers, are addressed by managing the symptoms, usually with drug therapy. Allopathic medicine does not seek to understand what causes most illness, and subsequently has no way of curing them. We have been conditioned to believe that this is state-of-the art medicine. How much money has been spent on research over the last thirty years with very few positive results? The price and amount of drugs being sold have increased drastically in the last ten years. Health care is costing us enormous amounts of money with little return on our investment. We keep looking down this straight and narrow path for the magic pill, not realizing that this quest is a mere illusion propagated by the pharmaceutical industry, and presented on a silver platter by the media. We all want the quick fix, no matter what the cost is down the road.

Symptoms only treated

Drugs are generally created to be taken on a daily basis for treating symptoms, not for curing diseases. You stop the drug and the symptoms return. The bottom line is profit, which is no different from fast food chains, tobacco companies or any other company. They are all publicly traded companies, which have a responsibility to their shareholders to maximize profits. If the drugs actually cured something, the patient would not need to buy any more pills. Profits would go down. This is called free enterprise, upon which our country is based.

Disease management is such an appropriate term for this way of treating illness. It is much more profitable than trying to find a cure. Drug approval is an expensive process. Pharmaceutical companies need to reap the harvest once the federal Food and Drug Administration (FDA) approves the drug. This way of practicing medicine has other ramifications. First, while the warning signs are being ignored, the cause of the patient's underlying condition can worsen. It is like your internal smoke alarm is going off daily, and you respond by pulling out the battery. Second, the drugs themselves not only can cause immediate reactions, but also can cause permanent damage down the line, often affecting other parts of the body, such as the liver and kidneys. This Band-Aid approach may have little relationship to what is actually causing the original problem.

How many times do we learn from the news that a drug once thought to be safe by the FDA has been pulled off the market? These reports do not account for all the unknown times that drugs cause secondary body malfunctions that lead to eventual diseases. These illnesses are not usually recognized or reported to be related to drugs that were taken even years earlier. I believe that this is much more common than the general public is aware of.

Research important

The bottom line is to do your own research. Question your doctor and get opinions from other health care practitioners. The patients who stand up to and question their doctor, as well as their alternative medicine doctors and practitioners, will have much more success with whatever therapy they decide is best for them. Research is vital, as it gives you the ability to make informed decisions. The worst words that can come out of your mouth are, "I'll do whatever you say, doctor."

References

Abramson, John, M.D. *Overdosed America: The Broken Promise of American Medicine*. New York: Harper Perennial, 2005.

Garritano, Joanna, M.D. "U.S. Health Care Puts Profit Over People," *Seattle Post-Intelligencer*, January 10, 2007.

Pugh, Tony. "Mediocre Doctoring the Norm," *The Denver Post*, March 18, 2006.

Moynihan, Ray and Alan Cassels. *Selling Sickness: How the World's Biggest Pharmaceutical Companies Are Turning Us All Into Patients*. New York: Nation Books, 2005.

Snyder Sachs, Jessica. "Are Antibiotics Killing Us?" *Discover*, November 2005.

"'Watch and Wait'–A Shift in Approach to Kids' Ear Infections," Pediatrics/Children's Health News, June 6, 2005.

Chapter 10: Nutritional Sensitivities Equal Nutritional Deficiencies

When the body is sensitive or allergic to a substance, that substance is then rejected on a cellular level by the body in terms of its ability to metabolize it. Any substance falls into this category. It may be a food substance, a nutrient or a brain chemical. Many of these are genetic sensitivities that can be passed on within the family.

Sensitivities important

When a patient tells me he is allergic to corn, then many times he is sensitive to vitamin A. This is because corn has an abundance of vitamin A. Wheat allergies also are common. An allergy to wheat usually means there is sensitivity to B complex. This does not mean that all of the individual vitamin Bs (such as B_6, B_{12} and folic acid) all are reactants. However, it usually means that some of these nutrients that we are ingesting on a regular basis can cause an immune reaction to occur within the body when they are ingested. This will add more internal stresses to the system. In both cases, the inability of these nutrients to metabolize causes a specific nutrient deficiency. Being deficient in vitamin A can lead to respiratory, skin, eye and immune system problems. A deficiency to several of the Bs can lead to neurological dysfunction such as depression, anxiety, sleep disorders, numbness and fatigue. B_6, B_{12} and folic acid deficiencies lead to blood deficiency/anemia. When the body is sensitive to a food substance, it also is sensitive to many of the components of that substance. Components of wheat are gluten, B complex as well as other nutrients. Wheat intolerance has its roots in these components. Iodine is an interesting mineral that has been overlooked despite its ability to upregulate the thyroid gland. Many thyroid problems are due to a lack of this very important nutrient. See Chapter 41: Thyroid Conditions.

This is not mainstream thinking, even in the alternative medicine world, as most people have been taught to believe that if you are deficient in a nutrient, then that particular deficiency should be addressed by taking more of it. I took many nutrients for years without noticing much of a change in how I felt. I took all the best vitamins that I could get into my system, but my body was not metabolizing them, so I received very little improvement in my symptoms. How many people are taking high doses of certain nutrients but come up lacking in those particular nutrients when tested? Taking a nutrient in foods or by pill makes no difference if the sensitivity exists. Your body will reject it on a cellular level and symptoms of that particular deficiency will continue to occur. Many common symptoms that we live with on a daily basis come from these types of sensitivities that do not allow the body to assimilate the vitamins and nutrients that it needs to function well.

Sensitivity repatterning

This is where sensitivity-repatterning techniques can make such a huge shift in how people can reduce and/or eliminate their reactions to certain substances as well as being able to assimilate those nutrients from substances. Sensitivity reactions can cause immune reactions. This creates much internal stress. Reducing and/or eliminating this stress allows for a much better functioning immune system. Being able to assimilate nutrients is the key to proper body functioning. The bottom line is that eating well and taking proper supplements does not always equate to proper assimilation and good health. See www.richbrightheart.com for more information on how this process works.

References

Brownstein, David, M.D. *Iodine: Why You Need It, Why You Can't Live Without It*. West Bloomfield, Michigan: Medical Alternatives Press, 2006.

Brownstein, David, M.D. *Overcoming Thyroid Disorders*. West Bloomfield, Michigan: Medical Alternatives Press, 2004.

Cutler, Ellen W., D.C. *Winning the War Against Asthma and Allergies: A Drug-Free Cure for Asthma and Allergy Sufferers*. Albany, New York: Delmar Publishers, 1998.

Leviton, Richard. "Say Goodbye to Allergies," *Alternative Medicine*, May 1999.

Weber, Linda. "Food Allergies," *Natural Health*, July-August 1998.

Chapter 11: Antioxidants and Phytonutrients

Phytonutrients and antioxidants are some of the most powerful natural substances that assist the body in reducing inflammation and free radicals They also support natural immune system functioning and prevent illness, according to extensive current research.

The role of antioxidants

Antioxidants neutralize free radicals by donating one of their own electrons. Electrons are negatively charged particles that surround an atom. They are involved in chemical reactions and are the substance that bonds atoms together to form molecules. Free radicals are unpaired electrons that break off and attack healthy tissue causing cellular damage. This damage increases under many conditions such as smoking, drugs, poor nutritional intake, alcohol, chronic infections, stress and long-term illnesses. This damage can lead to premature aging as well as many chronic conditions such as heart disease, strokes, both elevated and oxidized LDL cholesterol, cancer, diabetes and other chronic inflammatory conditions (PubMed Central, March 13, 2008). Numerous studies report that antioxidants can greatly reduce this process when ingested in various forms (Palan, January 1996; Abahusain, August 1999; McMillan, 2000; McMillan, 2002; and Randall, August 2, 2007).

The role of phytonutrients

Phytonutrients are chemical compounds that come from edible plants. In plants, protective self-repairing cell production is stimulated by phytonutrients. In humans, they produce the same kinds of responses. Many phytonutrients can be extracted from various fruits and natural substances. These compounds have been and are currently being studied for the purpose of supporting immune function, preventing illness, slowing the aging process and helping to support the body in healing. They are known for their strong antioxidant/free radicalsscavenging action as well as their ability to reduce inflammation. Phytonutrients are currently being studied in several arenas including cancer therapy, diabetes, cardiovascular disease and macular degeneration with some very positive results. The key sources of phytonutrients are berries, cruciferous and dark leafy vegetables, soy and red wine.

Some of the berries that seem to hold these properties include cranberries, blueberries, strawberries, goji berries, the palm berry acai and raspberries. In a recent study reported in the *American Journal of Clinical Nutrition*, seventy-two middle-age subjects with cardiovascular risk factors consumed moderate amounts of various berries for an eight-week, single-blind, randomized, placebo-controlled trial. The study concluded that the subjects achieved favorable changes in platelet function, HDL cholesterol and blood pressure. The results indicate that regular consumption of berries may play a significant role in the prevention of cardiovascular disease (Erlund, February 2008). Other key fruits include mangoes, pomegranates and noni fruit. One of the best examples is from research being done on a substance called ellagic acid, which is found in many fruits. The highest concentrations are in red raspberries and pomegranates.

Research at the Hollings Cancer Institute showed that ellagic acid is one of the most promising chemopreventative compounds discovered to date (CentreForce, April 13, 2007). It found antioxidant, antibacterial, antimutagenic, anticarcinogenic and antiviral properties.

Ellagic acid

The Hollings Institute states that ellagic acid promotes natural cell death of cervical cancer cells (Ellagic.net, 2003). It has similar effects on breast, pancreas, esophageal, skin, colon and prostate cancer cells, and it promotes wound healing (Ellagic.net, September 8, 2008 and Aviram, 2002). It works to quench molecules that oxidate, or add oxygen to cellular and circulatory proteins and fats, altering their biological function (EurekAlert, 2005). It also preserves circulating nitric oxide. Because of its anti-inflammatory and antioxidant capabilities, ellagic acid is a natural fit in supporting the body in cholesterol and other cardiovascular-related concerns as well as a host of other chronic conditions, according to studies.

Pomegranate juice

Pomegranate juice has been used since ancient times in the Middle East, Iran and India for treating disease and infection (Aviram, 2004). It is rich in tannins, phenolic and ellagic acid, polyphenols and flavonoids. It has been receiving significant attention due to recent studies that point to its characteristics as a strong antioxidant and anti-inflammatory agent. Research suggests that pomegranate may play a supportive role in suppressing tumor growth (EurekAlert, 2005; Jeune, Winter 2005; Harvard Men's Health Watch, April 1, 2007; Seeram, January 30, 2007; and American Technion Society, October 24, 2008). This supportive role could lead to cancer prevention and reduction, especially in breast and prostate cancer, as well as other prostate problems including the reduction in PSA levels (EurekAlert, 2005). Pomegranate juice can have positive benefits for erectile dysfunction, due to its increased blood flow and antioxidant properties (Newswise, August 24, 2005 and

DentalPlans, July 29, 2007). In cardiovascular disorders, pomegranate juice significantly reduced oxygen deficiency to the heart during exercise for patients with ischemic heart disease (DentalPlans, July 29, 2007). This indicated that blood flow to the heart was increased. A study also has shown it can reduce arterial plaque by 30 percent (Rosenblat, August 2006 and DentalPlans, July 29, 2007). Pomegranate juice also slows down cholesterol oxidation and minimizes the retention and aggregation of LDL cholesterol (Aviram, 2002; Nigris, March 1, 2005; and Rosenblat, August 2006). It may also reduce the plaque in arteries where there is heavy plaque buildup.

A study of forty-five patients with coronary heart disease with reduced blood flow to the heart was conducted by the Preventative Medicine Research Institute at the University of California at San Francisco and the California Pacific Medical Center. It showed that blood flow to the heart increased 17 percent after three months of drinking 8 ½ ounces of pomegranate juice a day (Sumner, September 15, 2005). The study also found the group that didn't drink pomegranate juice worsened by 18 percent. This showed a 35 percent difference between the two groups.

Another study was done by Professor Michael Aviram of the Lipid Research Lab at Rambam Medical Center in Haifa, Israel (Aviram, 2004). Nineteen patients with severe carotid artery narrowing were chosen. Ten of these received 8.3 ounces of pomegranate juice daily for one year while the other nine received a placebo. After one year, those consuming the pomegranate juice showed a 35 percent decrease of thickness in the carotid artery. Additionally, systolic blood pressure was reduced from 174 to 152. They also showed a reduction in oxidized cholesterol levels. The placebo group showed a 9 percent increase in carotid artery thickness.

Another study, conducted at the Technion-Israel Institute of Technology, was published in the May 2000 issue of the *American Journal of Clinical Nutrition* (Aviram, 2000). Subjects who drank two to three ounces of pomegranate juice per day for two weeks slowed cholesterol oxidation by as much as 40 percent. In the same study, mice showed a 44 percent reduction in legions within the arteries compared to the control group when fed pomegranate juice (Aviram, 2000).

What this proves is that pomegranate has the ability to severely reduce oxidative stress, which in turn lowers inflammation thereby reducing carotid artery thickness and improving antioxidant blood levels. It also has been shown to improve sperm quality in rats. Other studies have been done on mice showing positive cardiovascular benefits (Aviram, 2002 and Nigris, March 1, 2005). This potent reduction in both inflammation and oxidative stress is the key to lowering the risks of heart attacks, strokes and bad cholesterol. The future should see many more larger-scale studies due to the promising results already seen.

Raspberries, blueberries, cranberries, mangoes, goji berry, noni fruit and acai berries

Raspberries have the highest levels of ellagic acid. They are a great source for this key health promoting substance. Recent medical tests have shown that the red raspberry is one of the most effective all-natural ways to fight certain forms of cancer, according to Daniel Nixon, M.D., researcher from the Medical University of South Carolina (Centreforce, January 18, 2009).

Blueberries have shown to be beneficial as an antioxidant and for urinary tract infections, eyesight improvement, cholesterol control and anti-aging (World's Healthiest Foods, April 13, 2007 and Weekend Gardener, August 8, 2007). The key antioxidant components in blueberries are anthocyanin and cholenergenic acid. In a recent study reported in the *Journal of Nutritional Biochemistry*, rats that were fed blueberries daily for three months significantly increased their bone density (Wright, July/August 2008). "We believe that polyphenols in the berries slowed the rate [of bone turnover], ultimately saving bone," Bahram Arjmandi, Ph.D., the study's lead author and professor and chair of the department of nutrition, food and exercise sciences at Florida State University, said in an article about the study in *Eating Well* magazine.

Cranberries are most known for supporting urinary tract health. PACs are compounds in cranberries that are responsible for disabling harmful bacteria in the urinary system (News Target, April 13, 2007). They also help to remove bacteria from the lining.

Mangoes contain significant amounts of phytonutrients known as xanthones. Mangoes are high in antioxidants, and research has shown the fruit to have properties that support reducing inflammation as well as a healthy cardiovascular system.

Goji berries have nineteen amino acids including all eight essential amino acids (Goji Juice, August 8, 2007). They are high in carotenoids and contain beta-sitosterol, an anti-inflammatory agent. Goji berries also have twenty-one trace minerals and are a source of B vitamins and essential fatty acids.

Noni fruit has been used for centuries in Tahiti and Southeast Asia as a medicinal remedy for numerous conditions. Research shows that it helps stimulate the production of T-cells in the immune system (Solomon, November 1999). T-cells play a major role in immune health. Noni can also be used for antibacterial and antiseptic purposes. It contains seventeen of the twenty amino acids including eight essential amino acids.

Acai berries are a powerful superfood from the Amazon Rainforest. Acai berries are known for their high antioxidant properties (Amherst College, April 13, 2007). They contain chemicals called phenols and anthocyanin. Acai berries are packed with antioxidants, Omega-3 and Omega-6 fatty acids, B vitamins, calcium and phosphorus (Amazon Berry, April 13, 2007).

When people understand the positive impact that phytonutrients from these fruits can have on their overall health, it is an easy decision to begin daily supplementation. Taking a wide range of phytonutrients is the best approach. A supplement that I take daily contains a mixture of several of the key fruit sources listed above.

Resveratrol

Resveratrol is a polyphenol compound that is found in the skins of red grapes, which is often associated with the health benefits of red wine because of its powerful antioxidant and cardiovascular protection properties. Much has been written about this life-changing nutrient. A new research study on mice has shown additional properties that could increase the production of mitochondria (slender rods that are the source of cell energy), which can support a boosting of the metabolism. Resveratrol also has been shown to increase stamina and slow the aging process and may prevent certain diseases including heart disease, cancer and diabetes, according to studies. Resveratrol can support the overall health of the body and may help increase fat-burning metabolism (ScienceDaily, July 9, 2004). The good news is you do not have to be a wine drinker to reap the benefits as it is now being produced in capsule form.

Fortune magazine did a cover feature extolling the virtues of resveratrol's potential health benefits (Stipp, February 23, 2007). *Men's Journal, Best Life, The New York Times* and even the National Cancer Institute have written articles about its potential for protection from heart disease, diabetes, cancer, Alzheimer's disease and aging. This is why the French have such low levels of heart disease compared to Americans despite eating a high fat diet.

Resveratrol is also found in a plant called polygonum cuspidatum. This plant has been used in traditional Asian medicine in heart and liver medicines. Resveratrol scavenges the free radicals that oxidize cholesterol. In a study on mice, it was shown to improve their sensitivity to insulin. Resveratrol is a very small molecule that can penetrate the cell wall and enter the nucleus. Once inside, it can switch off genes that can initiate the progression of disease. It helps to block the replication of various pathogens as well as tumor cells (ScienceDaily, September 1, 2007 and Mitchell, April 16, 2008).

Resveratrol contributes to increased levels of the enzyme called SIRT1. This enzyme has been linked to longevity, DNA repair and insulin secretion. It also has been shown to improve insulin sensitivity. Resveratrol is known to activate the SIRT1 enzyme. This enzyme is decreased in insulin resistance cells and tissue. By supplementing with only 2.5 milligrams a day of resveratrol, enhanced insulin sensitivity to cells occurred, even under insulin resistant conditions (ScienceDaily, October 4, 2007).

The amount of resveratrol in red wine is very low, so people should not try to get this nutrient from wine. Drinking alcohol is not healthy on a regular basis. Supplementation is necessary for optimizing therapeutic levels of resveratrol. The amount that should be taken on a daily basis for meeting these levels needs to be determined. More long-term studies need to be done on what conditions can benefit from resveratrol and how much is indicated for therapeutic levels.

Green algae, barley grass, chlorella and spirulina

Various forms of green algae such as blue-green algae, barley grass, spirulina and chlorella have nutritional and immune supporting properties.

Algae such as blue green algae, spirulina and especially chlorella all support the body in detoxifying various chemicals and heavy metals. Algae contain significant amounts of various key nutrients.

Barley grass is very alkalizing, has detoxification qualities and is a great source of dense nutrition. It can be found in both powder and pill form.

Green tea

Green tea has many medicinal qualities. It has been used in Japan for years for various ailments.

Green tea contains significant amounts of flavonoids, quercetin and catechins. Quercetin is a flavonoid, and research shows that it has strong anti-inflammatory and anticancer properties. The key catechin found in green tea is epigallocatechin (EGCG). It is a strong antioxidant, and studies show EGCG plays a strong role in supporting the body in the prevention and reduction of various forms of cancer (Carter, June 2007 and Ogasawara, 2007). Green tea and its components seem to slow the development of cancer by suppressing the signals needed for cancer cell progression (Ohishi, January 27, 1997; Isemura, 2000; and Kuo, 2003). It also helps to block enzymes and proteins that are needed for tumor development. These studies show beneficial effects for many forms of cancer including colon, breast, prostate, bladder, ovarian, lung, pancreatic, rectal and skin cancer (Ji, January 27, 1997 and Arts, May 2002). Research includes both animal and human subjects.

EGCG also can improve cardiovascular function. It does this primarily by helping to decrease inflammation and oxidative stress. This in turn reduces the oxidation of LDL cholesterol (Vinson, 1995; Ishikawa, 1997; and Hofmann, April 2003). LDL cholesterol in an oxidized form is the number one factor involved in creation of heart attacks, strokes and atherosclerosis, according to research. EGCG also supports the body in increasing blood flow and lowering blood pressure by relaxing the arteries.

Green tea inhibits oxidative changes within the body caused from free radicals, pathogens and various carcinogens. It helps to inhibit the growth of abnormal cells by inhibiting the rate of how cells divide.

Green tea can greatly enhance immune function. Taken on a daily basis, its antioxidants and nutrients are custom made for supporting key components of the body by helping to enhance how the body functions at a cellular level.

The best way to receive the full benefits of green tea is to drink it in a specially prepared powdered form. In this form, nutrients are fully utilized by the body. Most people are not aware that more than 95 percent of the nutrients and antioxidants are left in the tea bag or tea leaves. Consuming the edible powdered form of green tea gives you 100 percent of the nutrients and antioxidants. Sencha is a form of green tea that has the highest antioxidants (Randall, August 2, 2007).

Studies on antioxidants

The following antioxidants have been subjected to numerous studies over many years. The key antioxidants are vitamins A (retinol), C, E (alpha-tocopherol) and beta-carotene; the minerals selenium and zinc; coenzyme Q10; lipoic acid, lycopene, lutein and zeaxanthin; essential fatty acids, such as omega-3 and omega-6; and bioflavanoids. When people combine antioxidants/phytonutrients into their daily food intake, current research shows that these nutrients may support the body in providing the appropriate building blocks for disease prevention as well as supporting their systems with whatever healing modalities they want to incorporate for any ill condition.

Consistent studies have shown that higher rates of antioxidant levels are related to lower C-reactive protein levels, a marker of inflammation, which translates to lower inflammation (Curran, 2000; McMillan, 2000; and *JACS*, July 2004). Lower inflammation means lower rates of many illnesses, such as cancer, diabetes and heart disease.

Sources of antioxidants

Coenzyme Q10 has been used in Europe for years as a main treatment for heart disease because it can help to strengthen the heart. It supports the body in increasing cellular energy. It helps the body utilize oxygen more effectively and supports immune function. High amounts of this nutrient are used by the heart to function to properly. Statin drugs lower coenzyme Q10 levels in the body, according to research studies.

Vitamin C is a strong antioxidant and has been known for years to have beneficial effects for immune function. Many people who take large doses of vitamin C at the onset of a cold claim to be able to ward off the cold. Recently, vitamin C has been studied for its anti-inflammatory capabilities. ScienceDaily on November 14, 2008, reported on a new study by researchers at the University of California at Berkeley showing evidence that vitamin C supplements have the ability to lower concentrations of C-reactive protein. A daily dose of vitamin C lowered the levels of the inflammation biomarker after two months for the participants with elevated C-reactive protein levels compared to those who took a placebo. More studies in this area would be beneficial in determining the impact of vitamin C on cardiovascular disease as well as other illnesses (ScienceDaily, November 14, 2008).

Lipoic acid is being investigated for its ability to reduce oxidative stress and chelate heavy metals (Zhang, March 13, 2008). It has been used for thirty years in Europe to prevent and treat complications associated with diabetes.

Flax seeds and chia seeds and their oils are very high in omega fatty acids. They are high in antioxidants, support immune function and help to reduce inflammation (OsteoarthritisRemedy, March 13, 2008).

Carotenoids (alpha-carotene, beta-carotene, beta-cryptoxanthin, lycopene and lutein/zeaxanthin) have shown a direct relationship to C-reactive protein levels (Kritchevsky, December 2000). The higher the blood carotenoid levels, the lower the C-reactive protein marker (Kritchevsky, December 2000). This shows that carotenoids have definite anti-inflammatory properties. Lycopene is found in tomato products and has strong antioxidant properties (Tyssandier, August 1, 2005). It has been shown to be beneficial as a protective agent against cancer, heart disease and macular degeneration. This is one of the main reasons the Mediterranean diet is so healthy (Olmedilla, 2001). Lutein and zeaxanthin are the only carotenoids present in the lens of the eye. Zeaxanthin is the dominate component in the macula and lutein is present throughout the retina.

Generally, the higher the antioxidant levels the lower the C-reactive protein levels. Higher levels of C-reactive protein are directly related to much higher rates of cardiovascular disease, cancer, diabetes, arthritis, pancreatitis and death, according to studies. This shows that the higher the inflammation, the more likely that people are to develop one of these or other major illnesses. Antioxidants lower C-reactive protein levels and oxidative stress. Studies have shown that a strong relationship exists between higher intakes of these nutrients, which help to raise circulating antioxidant levels, and lower rates of the above illnesses and other major illnesses as well (Palan, January 1996; Abahusain, August 1999; van Campenhout, November/December 2006; Mitchell, March 13, 2008; and PubMed, March 13, 2008). We can clearly see the positive benefits of taking them. These results are from an accumulation of many studies over a period of time that consistently show this correlation. Just think how healthy our country would be if we embraced this knowledge. People need to seek out health information for themselves as the traditional medical community and the drug-promoting media are not inclined to inform you.

Fish oil

Omega-3 fatty acids are a group of lipid compounds (OsteoarthritisRemedy, March 13, 2008). The two most important omega-3 fatty acids are DHA and EPA. The body needs EPA in order to produce series 3 prostaglandins. These are hormone-like substances that have positive effects on blood pressure, cholesterol, triglyceride levels, kidney function, immune response, reproduction and inflammation.

Fish oil is high in omega-3 fatty acids. It is believed to have anti-inflammatory properties, thereby promoting heart health and preventing oxidative stress. Fish oil produces chemicals called resolvins. These natural chemicals play a strong role in reducing the inflammatory process. Resolvins act to stop the migration of inflammatory cells to the injury sites. They also decrease the formation of chemicals called prostanoids, which promote leukotriene and cox-1 and cox-2 proinflammatory mediators. This differs from cox-2 inhibitor types of drugs, which can be damaging to the heart. In contrast, fish oil is naturally good for the heart.

Fish oil is essential for the health of the eyes as well as the nervous and reproductive systems (Spectacle World, March 13, 2008). It has been extensively researched as having positive benefits in arthritis, inflammatory bowel disease and

Alzheimer's. It has other wonderful benefits as well including improved cognitive function, mood and memory enhancement, increased blood flow, vascular relaxation, healthy triglycerides, visual improvements and macular health. Fish oil also supports the body's ability to enhance proanti-inflammatory prostaglandins and reduce proinflammatory cytokines, according to research studies (Arita, March 2007; Wade, August 2007; and Galarrage, March 2008).

Antioxidant and phytonutrients supplements

It is difficult to get all these beneficial nutrients at the proper levels without supplementation. Whole food supplements contain significant amounts of these ingredients. Many can be taken in pill form, but they also can be found in powder form. Powders often save people money, and they can be incorporated into a morning smoothie. The berry nutrients are best eaten in their natural form as well as taken in pill or powder form. I suggest people avoid juices, if possible, due to high sugar levels in the juice. Many juices on the market contain less vital and essential types of juice. Even if the juice product is labeled pomegranate juice, it may contain very little pomegranate juice and high amounts of less costly fillers such as apple and orange juice. These fillers are high in sugar and lower in key nutrient density. This is a problem for people who are trying to lose weight or have *Candida albicans* or blood sugar regulation issues.

Antioxidants and phytonutrients are so powerful that I think they should be added to our water supply. By examining all the legitimate research that has been done on antioxidants in the last ten years, a correlation can be observed between adding the proper amounts of these nutrients to the daily diet and the reduction of cardiovascular disease, cancer and a host of other diseases. Phytonutrients and antioxidants are the key to a healthier and happier life. Research suggests that the more people take, the healthier they will become and the less chance they will have for any illness to take hold.

Notes

Abahusain, M.A. et al. "Retinol, Alpha-Tocopherol and Carotenoids in Diabetes," *European Journal of Clinical Nutrition*, August 1999.

"Acai: Nature's Energy Fruit," Amazon Berry, Accessed April 13, 2007. www.amazonberry.com.au/the_acai_story.php

"The Amazing Amazon Rainforest," Amherst College, Accessed April 13, 2007. www.amherst.edu/~dmirwin/aciareport.htm

"Antioxidants for Inflammation," OsteoarthritisRemedy.com, Accessed March 13, 2008. www.osteoarthritisremedy.com/herbal-remedies/inflammationremedy/antioxidants-for-inflammation

"Antioxidant Supplement Use Associated With Lower Inflammatory Markers," *Journal of the American Geriatrics Society*, July 2004.

"Antioxidants," Spectacle World, Accessed March 13, 2008. www.spectacleworld.co.za/eyehealth.htm

Arita, Makoto, M.D. "Stereochemical Assignment, Anti-inflammatory Properties, and Receptor for the Omega-3 Lipid Mediator Resolvin E-1," *Journal of Experimental Medicine*, March 2007.

Arts, I.C. et al. "Dietary Catechins and Cancer Incidence Among Postmenopausal Women: The Iowa Women's Health Study," *Cancer Causes Control*, May 2002.

Aviram, M. et al. "Pomegranate Juice Consumption for Three Years by Patients With Carotid Artery Stenosis Reduces Common Carotid Intima-media Thickness, Blood Pressure, and LDL Oxidation," *Clinical Nutrition*, Vol. 3, Issue 3, 2004.

Aviram, M. et al. "Pomegranate Juice Consumption Reduces Oxidative Stress, Atherogenic Modifications to LDL, and Platelet Aggregation: Studies in Humans and in Atherosclerotic Apolipoprotein E-deficient Mice," *The American Journal of Clinical Nutrition*, May 2000.

Aviram, M. et al. "Pomegranate Juice Flavonoids Inhibit Low-Density Lipoprotein Oxidation and Cardiovascular Diseases: Studies in Atherosclerotic Mice and in Humans," *Drugs Under Experimental and Clinical Research*, Issue 2-3, 2002.

"The Amazing Amazon Rainforest," Amherst College, Accessed April 13, 2007. www.amherst.edu/~dmirwin/AcaiReport.htm

"Benefits of Blueberries," Weekend Gardener, Accessed August 8, 2007.
www.weekendgardener.net/medicinal-plants/benefits-of-blueberry-juice-60601.htm

"Blueberries," World's Healthiest Foods, Accessed April 13, 2007.
www.whfoods.com/genpage.php?tname=foodspice&dbid=8

"Can Pomegranates Prevent Prostate Cancer? A New Study Offers Promise,"
EurekAlert, 2005, Accessed July 28, 2007.
www.eurekalert.org/pub_releases/2005-09/uow-cpp092205.php

Canene-Adams, K. et al. "Collective Phytochemical Activity of Whole Tomato and
Broccoli Significantly More Effective in Slowing Prostate Tumor Growth than
Lycopene Alone," *Cancer Research*, Vol. 67, No. 2, 2007.

Carter, O. et al. "Comparison of White Tea, Green Tea, Epigallocatechin-3-gallate,
and Caffeine as Inhibitors of PhIP-Induced Colonic Aberrant Crypts," *Nutrition and
Cancer*, June 2007.

"Cranberries Show Remarkable Health Benefits in Studies," News Target, Accessed
April 13, 2007.
www.newstarget.com/021168.html

Curran, F. et al. "Relationship of Carotenoids and Vitamins A and E With the Acute
Inflammatory Response in Acute Pancreatitis," *British Journal of Surgery*, Vol. 87, Issue
3, 2000.

"Dietary Intakes and Plasma Concentrations of Carotenoids and Tocopherols in
Relation to Glucose Metabolism in Subjects at High Risk of Type 2 Diabetes: the
Botina Dietary Study," PubMed, National Institutes of Health, Accessed March 13,
2008.
www.ncbi.nlm.nih.gov/pubmed/12791620

"Ellagic Acid," Centreforce, Accessed April 13, 2007.
health.centreforce.com/health/berries.html

"Ellagic Acid–Clinical Studies," Ellagic.net, Accessed September 8, 2008.
www.ellagic.net/ellagic-acid-clinical studies.html

"Ellagic Acid May Be One of the Most Potent Ways to Prevent Cancer," Ellagic.net, 2003, Accessed September 8, 2008. www.ellagic.net/ellagic-acid-background.html

"Ellagic Acid–Medical References," Ellagic.net, 2003, Accessed September 8, 2008. www.ellagic.net/ellagic-acid-medical-references.html

Erlund, Iris. "Favorable Effects of Berry Consumption on Platelet Function, Blood Pressure, and HDL Cholesterol," *American Journal of Clinical Nutrition*, February 2008.

"Fish Oil and Inflammation," OsteoarthritisRemedy.com, Accessed March 13, 2008. www.osteoarthritisremedy.com/herbal-remedies/inflammationremedy/fish-oil-and-inflammation

Galarrage, B. et al. "Cod Liver Oil (n-3 Fatty Acids) as an Non-Steroidal Anti-Inflammatory Drug Sparing Agent in Rheumatoid Arthritis," *Rheumatology*, March 2008.

"Health Benefits of Pomegranate Juice," DentalPlans, Accessed July 29, 2007. www.dentalplans.com/Dental-Health-Articles/Health-benefits-of-pomegranate-juice.asp

"Health Benefits and Pomegranate Juice," Newswise Medical News, August 24, 2005, Accessed October 24, 2008. www.newswise.com/articles/view/51398/

Hofmann, C.S. and G.E. Sonenshein. "Green Tea Polyphenol Epigallocatechin-3-gallate Induces Apoptosis of Proliferating Vascular Smooth Muscle Cells via Activation of p53," *FASEB Journal*, April 2003.

Isemura, M. et al. "Tea Catechins and Related Polyphenols as Anti-Cancer Agents," *Biofactors*, Vol. 13, No. 1-4, 2000.

Ishikawa, T. et al. "Effect of Tea Flavonoid Supplementation on the Susceptibility of Low-density Lipoprotein to Oxidative Modification," *American Journal of Clinical Nutrition*, Issue 66, 1997.

Jeune, M.A. et al. "Anticancer Activities of Pomegranate Extracts and Genistein in Human Breast Cancer Cells," *Journal of Medicinal Food*, Winter 2005.

Ji, B.T. et al. "Green Tea Consumption and the Risk of Pancreatic and Colorectal Cancers," *International Journal of Cancer*, January 27, 1997.

Kritchevsky, S.B. et al. "Serum Carotenoids and Markers of Inflammation in Nonsmokers," *American Journal of Epidemiology*, December 2000.

Kuo, P.L. and C.C. Lin. "Green Tea Constituent (-)-Epigallocatechin-3-gallate Inhibits HepG2 Cell Proliferation and Induces Apoptosis Through p53-dependent and Fas-mediated Pathways," *Journal of Biomedical Science*, Vol. 10, No. 2, 2003.

"Lower Concentrations of Carotenoids in the Critically Ill Patient Are Related to Systemic Inflammatory Response and Increased Lipid Peroxidation," PubMed, National Institutes of Health, Accessed March 13, 2008. www.ncbi.nlm.nih.gov/pubmed/14512033

McMillan, D. et al. "Changes in Micronutrient Concentrations Following Anti-Inflammatory Treatment in Patients With Gastrointestinal Cancer," *Nutrition*, Vol. 16, Issue 6, 2000.

McMillan, D. et al. "The Relationship Between Reduced Vitamin Antioxidant Concentrations and the Systemic Inflammatory Response in Patients With Common Solid Tumors," *Clinical Nutrition*, Vol. 21, Issue 2, 2002.

Mitchell, Terri. "Antioxidants," *Life Extension*, Accessed March 13, 2008. www.lef.org/magazine/mag2005/aug2005_report_antiox_03.htm

Mitchell, Terri. "Resveratrol: Cutting-Edge Technology Available Today," *Life Extension*, Accessed April 16, 2008. www.lef.org/LEFCMS/aspx/PrintVersionMagic.aspx?CmsID=110869

"More Medical Research Confirms Eating Red Raspberries May Be One of the Most Potent Ways to Fight Cancer," Centreforce, Accessed January 18, 2009. www.prostatecanceralternatives.com/Raspberry%20Red%20Raspberries.htm

Nigris, F. et al. "Beneficial Effects of Pomegranate Juice on Oxidation-Sensitive Genes and Endothelial Nitric Oxide Synthase Activity at Sites of Perturbed Shear Stress," *Proceedings of the National Academy of Sciences*, March 21, 2005.

"Nutritional Antioxidants and the Modulation of Inflammation: Theory and Practice," PubMed Central, National Institutes of Health, Accessed March 13, 2008. www.ncbi.nlm.nih.gov/pubmed/7922442

Ogasawara, M. et al. "Differential Effects of Antioxidants on the In Vitro Invasion, Growth and Lung Metastasis of Murine Colon Cancer Cells," Biological and Pharmaceutical Bulletin, Vol. 30, No. 1, 2007.

Ohishi, T. et al. "Synergistic Effects of (-)-Epigallocatechin Gallate With Sulindac Against Colon Carcinogenesis of Rats Treated With Azoxymethane," *Cancer Letter*, January 27, 1997.

Olmedilla, B. et al. "Serum Concentrations of Carotenoids and Vitamins A, E, and C in Control Subjects From Five European Countries," *British Journal of Nutrition*, Vol. 85, 2001.

Palan, P.R. et al. "Plasma Levels of Beta-Carotene, Lycopene, Canthaxanthin, Retinol, and Alpha- and Tau-tocopherol in Cervical Intraepithelial Neoplasia and Cancer," *Clinical Cancer Research*, Vol. 2, January 1996.

"Pomegranate Juice May Be Good for the Prostate and Heart, Reports the Harvard Men's Health Watch," Harvard Health Publications, April 1, 2007, Accessed October 24, 2008. www.health.harvard.edu/press_releases/health-benefits-of-pomegranate-juice

"Pomegranate Juice Slows PSA Acceleration Rate After Prostate Cancer Surgery, Radiation," EurekAlert, Accessed July 29, 1997. www.eurekalert.org/pub_releases/2006-07/aafc-pjs062706.php

"Pomegranate Seed Oil Causes Breast Cancer Cells to Self-Destruct," American Technion Society, Accessed October 24, 2008. www.ats.org/news.php?id=32

"Prospective Study of Carotenoids, Tocopherols, and Retinoid Concentrations and the Risk of Breast Cancer," PubMed, National Institutes of Health, Accessed March 13, 2008.
www.ncbi.nlm.nih.gov/pubmed/12010859

Randall, Barb. "Use Antioxidants (Have I Ever Steered You Wrong?)," *Lake Oswego Review/West Linn Tidings*, August 2, 2007.

"Red Wine Compound Shown to Prevent Prostate Cancer," ScienceDaily, September 1, 2007.
www.sciencedaily.com/releases/2007/08/070831131320.htm

"Red Wine Ingredient—Resveratrol—Fights Diabetes in Mice," ScienceDaily, October 4, 2007.
www.sciencedaily.com/releases/2007/10/071002131152.htm

"The Risk of Developing Lung Cancer Associated With Antioxidants in the Blood: Ascorbic Acid, Carotenoids, Alpha-Tocopherol, Selenium, and Total Peroxyl Radical Absorbing Capacity," PubMed, National Institutes of Health, Accessed March 13, 2008.
www.ncbi.nlm.nih.gov/pubmed/9367064

Rosenblat, Mira et al. "Anti-Oxidative Effects of Pomegranate Juice Consumption by Diabetic Patients on Serum and on Macrophages," *Atherosclerosis*, August 2006.

Seeram, N.P. et al. "Pomegranate Ellagitannin-Derived Metabolites Inhibit Prostate Cancer Growth and Localize to the Mouse Prostate Gland," *Journal of Agricultural and Food Chemistry*, January 30, 2007.

Solomon, N., M.D. "Noni: Nature's Health-Enhancing Fruit," Positive Health, November 1999.

Stipp, David. "Drink Wine and Live Longer," *Fortune*, February 23, 2007.

"Study Identifies Genetics of Fat Metabolism, Red Wine Link," ScienceDaily, July 9, 2004.

www.sciencedaily.com/releases/2004/07/040709085724.htm

Sumner, M. et al. "Effects of Pomegranate Juice Consumption on Myocardial Perfusion in Patients With Coronary Heart Disease," *American Journal of Cardiology*, September 15, 2005.

Tyssandier, V. et al. "Effect of Tomato Product Consumption on the Plasma Status of Antioxidant Microconstituents and on the Plasma Total Antioxidant Capacity in Healthy Subjects," *Journal of the American College of Nutrition*, August 1, 2005.

van Campenhout, Ann et al. "Impact of Diabetes Mellitus on the Relationship Between Iron, Inflammatory, and Oxidative Stress Status," *Diabetes/Metabolism Research and Review*, Vol. 22, November/December 2006.

Vinson, J.A. et al. "Plant Flavonoids, Especially Tea Flavonols, Are Powerful Antioxidants Using an In Vitro Oxidation Model for Heart Disease," *Journal of Agriculture and Food Chemistry*, Issue 42, 1995.

"Vitamin C Lowers Levels of Inflammation Biomarker Considered Predictor of Heart Disease," ScienceDaily, November 14, 2008. www.sciencedaily.com/releases/2008/11/081113091630.htm

Wade, M. et al, "Enzymes and Receptors of Prostaglandin Pathways With Arachidonic Acid-Derived Versus Eicosapentaenoic Acid-Derived Substrate and Products," *Journal of Biological Chemistry*, August 2007.

"What Is Goji Juice," Goji Juice, Accessed August 8, 2007. www.gojiberryjuice.org

Wright, Brierley. "The Total-Body Benefits of Berries," *Eating Well*, July/August 2008.

Zhang, Weijian, M.D., Ph.D. "The Role of Lipoic Acid in Inflammation and Atherosclerosis," Linus Pauling Institute, Oregon State University. lpi.oregonstate.edu/ss03/lipoicacid.html

References

Abiaka, C.D. et al. "Plasma Micronutrient Antioxidant in Cancer Patients," *Cancer Detection and Prevention*, Vol. 25, Issue 3, 2001.

Almushatat, A. et al. "Vitamin Antioxidants, Lipid Peroxidation, and the Systematic Inflammatory Response in Patients With Prostate Cancer," *International Journal of Cancer*, Vol. 118, Issue 4.

Black, Evelyn I. et al. "Antioxidant Deficiency in Cystic Fibrosis: When Is the Right Time to Take Action?" *American Society for Clinical Nutrition*, August 2004.

Chang, C. et al. "Plasma Levels of Lipophilic Antioxidant Vitamins in Acute Ischemic Stroke Patients: Correlation to Inflammation Markers and Neurological Deficits," *Nutrition*, Vol. 21, Issue 10, 2005.

Erlinger, Thomas, M.D., et al. "Relationship Between Systemic Markers of Inflammation and Serum B-Carotene Levels," *Archives of Internal Medicine*, Vol. 161, 2001.

Ito, Y. et al. "Lung Cancer Mortality and Serum Levels of Carotenoids, Retinol, Tocopherols, and Folic Acid in Men and Woman: A Case-Control Study Nested in the JACC Study," *Journal of Epidemiology*, Vol. 15, Supplement II, 2005.

Ito, Y. et al. "Serum Antioxidants and Subsequent Mortality Rates of All Causes of Cancer Among Rural Japanese Inhabitants," *International Journal for Vitamin and Nutrition Research*, July 2002.

"Lipoic Acid May Fight Atherosclerosis, Weight Gain," *Life Extension*, May 2008.

"Lower Prostate Cancer Risk in Men With Elevated Plasma Lycopene Levels: Results of a Prospective Analysis," PubMed, National Institutes of Health, Accessed March 13, 2008.
www.ncbi.nlm.nih.gov/pubmed/10096552

"Lycopene, Beta-Carotene and Colorectal Adenomas," PubMed Central, National Institutes of Health, Accessed March 13, 2008.
www.ncbi.nlm.nih.gov/pubmed/14668286?ordinalpos=27&itool=EntrezSystem2.PE

"Lycopene Stops BPH in its Tracks," *Life Extension*, May 2008.

McMillian, Donald C. et al. "Measurement of the Systemic Inflammatory Response Predicts Cancer-Specific and Non-cancer Survival in Patients With Cancer," *Nutrition and Cancer*, September 2001.

Ozner, Michael, M.D. "Enhancing Longevity Through the Miami Mediterranean Diet," *Life Extension*, May 2008.

Schunemann, Holger J. et al. "The Relation of Serum Levels of Antioxidant Vitamins C and E, Retinol, and Carotenoids With Pulmonary Functions in the General Population," *American Journal of Respiratory and Critical Care Medicine*, April 2001.

Shin, Min-Jeong et al. "Relationship Between Insulin Resistance and Lipid Peroxidation and Antioxidant Vitamins in Hypercholesterolemic Patients," *Journal of Nutrition and Metabolic Diseases and Dietetics*, Vol. 50, No. 2, 2006.

Talwar, D. et al. "Effect of Inflammation on Measures of Antioxidant Status in Patients With Non-small Cell Lung Cancer," *American Journal of Clinical Nutrition*, November 1977.

Turk, G. et al. "Effects of Pomegranate Juice Consumption on Sperm Quality, Spermatogenic Cell Density, Antioxidant Activity and Testosterone Level in Male Rats," *Clinical Nutrition*, January 25, 2008.

"Vitamin E and Inflammation," OsteoarthritisRemedy.com, Accessed March 13, 2008. www.osteoarthritisremedy.com/herbal-remedies/inflammationremedy/vitamin-e-and-inflammation

Voorrips, Laura E. et al. "A Prospective Cohort Study on Antioxidant and Folate Intake and Male Lung Cancer Risk," *American Association for Cancer Research*, April 2000.

Chapter 12: Cleansing and Detoxification

At the beginning of the healing process, I work with patients on detoxifying their systems. The body is like a car; you have to change the filter. Otherwise, the car may wear out ahead of time.

Body cleansing

You can cleanse the body in many ways. Many people think that when I mention cleansing they must go on a fast and drink carrot juice all day, or consume some awful tasting and smelling concoction from a Chinese herb store. That would work, but it is not required. Many manufacturers of natural supplements that I work with have formulas specific to organ and lymph detoxification. The liver, kidneys and colon are the main organs of elimination. The colon is like a trash can; it must be cleaned out from time to time. You take the trash can outside, use soap and water and scrub until it looks like new again. What happens if we do not clean it out on a regular basis? Bacteria and dirt start to accumulate, and it begins to smell. Just imagine what goes on in some people's colons who eat a typical American diet. They have a great deal of compacted fecal matter within their colon. This fecal matter will back up, as it is constantly being recirculated throughout the system, placing a toxic strain on the liver, kidneys and lymph system. These organs must take the brunt of a toxic colon. The lungs and skin also support this process. They need help from time to time in order to keep up with the strain of the American lifestyle. They can get overloaded with toxins and function at a subpar state.

My brother, for instance, a motorcycle mechanic for decades, typically changes his oil ahead of time and always stresses to me the importance of clean oil. However, he eats the worst diet and somehow fails to make the connection between his poor polluted blood and engine oil. If your engine does not function well with worn out toxic oil, then what do you think is going on with the blood inside of your body? You can always buy a new car, but new bodies are in short supply.

I suggest specific formulas for each organ in order to cleanse them properly. I usually have people begin using liver, kidney, colon and lymphatic cleansers to start the detoxification process. The body can heal much easier when it is not in toxin overload. Sometimes the patient will start to feel better once this process gets underway. Cleansers usually come in pill or liquid form and can be taken once a day in the morning for a period of time until the system is cleansed.

Detoxification

Heavy metal detoxification can be more detailed and may need to be added to the program, if a person's system is being compromised in this area. Heavy metals such as lead, mercury, cadmium and other toxic metals, along with certain solvents and other chemicals, may be the cause of some autoimmune reactions, as well as internally poisoning the body.

Mercury fillings, vaccines and our toxic environment are the main culprits. Few people know that mercury has been used for years in vaccines as a preservative and can add to your chances of getting mercury toxicity. Think of all the older folks who get their yearly flu vaccine. How many children now get more than twenty mercury-ladened vaccines during the early brain developing years? Mercury has been implicated in attention deficit disorder and autism, as it is highly toxic to an infant's developing brain. I am amazed that there are dentists who are still putting mercury in patients' mouths. How much proof do we need before we wake up and start to do the right thing? The immune system sees mercury as an invader, so it will start attacking it much like a pathogen. It can settle in any body tissue, including the brain.

Cilantro, garlic, chlorella and reduced glutathione are some of the best heavy metal chelators available. Intravenous chelation therapy is another option for getting the heavy metals out of the system. Colonic irrigation is also an effective option for colon cleansing. Most people derive great benefits from this therapy. Colonics is a water enema that reaches all parts of the colon with much more force.

One of the most effective ways of detoxifying the entire system is to use a dry far infrared sauna. These portable saunas are able to draw toxins out through the pores. Using far infrared saunas on a regular basis for three to six months can result in a huge reduction in a person's toxic load. These units, formerly costing thousands of dollars, are now available in a portable unit for only a few hundred dollars.

Benefits of cleansing and detoxification

All these methods of cleansing and detoxification need to be part of the big picture in order to achieve long-term desired results. Another bonus is that it helps to prevent future illness, especially colon problems, as well as all types of cancers. Cleansing the body should be done at least twice a year for optimum health. If everyone did this as recommended, millions of dollars would be saved in our health care system, in addition to alleviating much suffering and saving lives. A clean internal environment is a low-cost investment, which pays high long-term dividends. See www.richbrightheart.com for more information on current nutritional protocols.

References

Cecchini, Marie A., M.S., David E. Root, M.D., M.P.H., Jeremie R. Rachunow, M.D., and Phyllis Gelb, M.D. "Chemical Exposures at the World Trade Center," *Townsend Letter for Doctors and Patients*, April 2006.

Foster, John S., M.D., Patricia C. Kane, Ph.D., and Neal Speight, M.D. "The Detoxx™ System: Detoxification of Biotoxins in Chronic Neurotoxic Syndromes," *Townsend Letter for Doctors and Patients*, November 2002.

Chapter 13: Antibiotics

In many ways antibiotics have done much good for our society. They solved the tuberculosis problem as well as many other infections. At that time there was no other way of treating these types of diseases. Antibiotics have saved many lives in these cases. They have come a long way in terms of what they can treat and how specific they can be for certain bacteria. Antibiotics still have a place in our medical system if used appropriately. I want you to understand the downside of antibiotics, because this can shed some light on when and when not to use them.

The antibiotic problem

Candida albicans has become epidemic in our society and is probably just as epidemic in other societies that use antibiotics so freely. Antibiotics were never meant to be used for convenience, such as having a cold, earache, sore throat or sinus infection. The body's immune system has the ability to overcome most acute colds. These other conditions are best treated in ways that do not compromise the immune system down the road. First, antibiotics suppress the immune function by not allowing your immune system to do its job. Secondly, repeated use of antibiotics disrupts the intestinal flora and its delicate balance. I do not think most people understand the consequences of this.

After you have taken antibiotics more than three times in your life, there is usually a permanent change of good bug to bad bug ratio in your intestinal tract. Why is this so important? Because once this balance is disturbed, your digestive and immune systems are altered forever. The intestinal ecosystem's checks and balances have shifted. *Candida albicans* is one of the bad bugs that takes over and overshadows the healthy gut microflora, which has been destroyed by the antibiotics. *Clostridium difficile*, another normal intestinal bacterium, can also become a virulent pathogen as it can get out of balance as well. When the intestinal balance is altered, it greatly lowers immune function. It does so because *Candida* is an invasive pathogen that can infest the whole body.

Antibiotic research

An article in the September 2005 issue of *Discover* magazine entitled, "Are Antibiotics Killing Us?" gave excellent facts to explain this growing problem. Microbiologist Abigail Salyers, at the University of Illinois, said her research shows that decades of antibiotic use have bred a frightening degree of drug resistance into our intestinal flora. She said that having a highly antibiotic-resistant bacterial population makes a person "a ticking time bomb." In the same article Infectious-disease Specialist Curtis Donskey, of Case Western University, said, "Unfortunately far too many physicians are still thinking of antibiotics as benign. We're just now beginning to understand how our normal microflora does such a good job of preventing colonization by disease causing microbes. We're just starting to understand the medical consequences of disturbing that with antibiotics." He also said that a nasty strain of *Clostridium difficile* has killed hundreds of hospital patients in Canada over the past two years, and this same strain is moving into hospitals in the United States (Snyder, November 2005).

An article in *The Olympian* newspaper dated December 31, 2005, entitled, "Mystery Intestinal Bug Striking More Patients," stated, "The increased use of antibiotics and heartburn drugs are to blame for the rise of bacterial infections." The article also said that *Clostridium difficile* appears to be spreading rapidly around the country causing unusually severe and sometimes fatal illness. Clifford McDonald of the federal Centers for Disease Control and Prevention in Atlanta said in the article, "We're very concerned. We know it is happening, but we are not sure why or where it is going" (Stein, December 31, 2005).

Any lingering pathogen will lower immune function depending upon what type of impact it is having on the immune system. Some of the research I have done indicates that *Candida* actually helps to fuel other pathogens, or possibly increase their virulence. Because it lowers immune function, it will be much easier to allow other pathogens to invade the system. Huge problems happen when there are multiple pathogens in the system, especially when they are being fueled by the *Candida*. Also, antibiotics cause bacteria and other pathogens to alter their cell wall structure in order to become more resistive. An article in the *Seattle Post-Intelligencer*, dated August 26, 2005, reported a study by scientists showing that bacteria can build a biofilm resistive wall around themselves in response to the presence of antibiotics. This was identified with the bacterium *Pseudomonas* that causes difficult-to-treat lung infections in people with cystic fibrosis. The study was done by the University of Washington and Rutgers University. Other researchers also have proven that the bacterium *Staphylococcus aureus* has similar biofilm building capabilities. The other key factor is how bacteria are altering their cell walls to be much more resistant and aggressive with the use of antibiotic therapy. Lastly, this altered intestinal environment sets the stage for leaky gut syndrome (*Seattle Post-Intelligencer*, August 25, 2005). See Chapter 15: Leaky Gut Syndrome and Chapter 19: Cell Wall Deficient Pathogens.

A long-term problem

When a patient gets a cold and immediately goes to the doctor to ask for antibiotics and the doctor denies the request, many patients feel that she is not a good doctor. Patients do not realize that they may be undermining their long-term health by taking antibiotics. It is a short-term fix that sets the stage for long-term problems. No one is policing the antibiotic industry, because antibiotics do not cause death directly. They, however, set in motion the building blocks for a slow degradation of overall health. They create so much long-term illness that often cannot be pinpointed back to the origination of taking the antibiotics. In my personal experience, it took me five or more years for my candida symptoms to get full blown. Had I not done my own research, I would have never suspected that taking tetracycline years earlier would have caused the horrible symptoms I had.

Almost every patient who I have seen in my practice that has been on repeated doses of antibiotics generally seems to have a multitude of physical problems at some point. In my experience, antibiotics should be used when there is a threat of death and, possibly, for certain needed surgeries. Dentists are requiring patients to take antibiotics to prevent bacterial infection, even in minor dental procedures. Children that are put on antibiotics early on for earaches actually have a higher incidence of recurrent ear infections than those who did nothing. This has been recently proven by several large-scale studies. Some of these studies also indicate that these same children also had much higher occurrences of allergies and asthma. (See Chapter 34: Ear and Eye Conditions.) The studies urged all pediatricians to be more prudent in their use of antibiotics. These studies were reported in mainstream newspapers, television news broadcasts and medical journals. This is again due to the antibiotics' ability to mutate the specific bacterium that causes the earache, and also the increased chance of getting *Candida albicans* from repeated doses, which lowers overall immune function, sometimes permanently.

Natural antibiotics

Alternatives are available that can function as natural antibiotics. The key is not to degrade the immune system, but to help build it. A strong immune system and healthy intestinal bacterial balance will then be able to ward off future predators, or at least help you to recover more quickly, so you do not have to rely on antibiotics. Ultimately, it is up to the patient to understand the potential long-term consequences of taking antibiotics. Information has been coming out for more than two decades, which, hopefully, has caught the eye of some allopathic physicians so that they understand that prudence in antibiotic use is what is most beneficial for their patients' long-term health.

The first book on this subject, *The Yeast Connection*, by William Crook, M.D., in the 1980s, became a best seller. His follow-up was entitled *The Yeast Connection and Chronic Fatigue Syndrome*. Since then, hundreds of articles and books have been written on this important subject. Patients come into my office and tell me how many times they have taken antibiotics. Many are still completely unaware of this ongoing danger, because no one has informed them about the repercussions of using antibiotics.

Educating patients is essential to their understanding that they need not use these drugs unless it is an absolute emergency. Herbs, such as Echinacea and goldenseal, as well as olive and oregano leaf extracts, garlic, zinc and vitamin C can help. Homeopathic formulas and Chinese herbs along with acupuncture are other options as they can help not only to ward off a cold, but also support the immune system in the process. There are immune system formulas that combine many of these ingredients for a synergistic effect. These substances function much like natural antibiotics, but do not destroy the good intestinal flora. Why should people start permanently degrading their health when there are healthy alternative options?

See my website www.richbrightheart.com for information on some of these options.

Notes

Paulson, Tom. "Antibiotics Prompt Bacteria 'Walls,'" *Seattle Post-Intelligencer,* August 25, 2005.

Snyder Sachs, Jessica. "Are Antibiotics Killing Us?" *Discover*, November 2005.

Stein, Rob. "Mystery Intestinal Bug Striking More Patients," *The Olympian*, December 31, 2005.

References

"Antibiotic Use in Infants May Double Asthma Risk," PR Newswire, March 16, 2006. www.prnewswire.com/cgi-bin/stories.pl?ACCT=104&STORY=/www/story/03-13-1281024

Crook, William G., M.D. *Chronic Fatigue Syndrome and the Yeast Connection*. Jackson, Tennessee: Professional Books, 1992.

Crook, William G., M.D. *The Yeast Connection*. Jackson, Tennessee: Professional Books, Third Edition, 1986-1989.

Deadman, Peter and Mazin Al-Khafaji. *A Manual of Acupuncture*. Vista, California: Eastland Press, 1998.

Gronczewski, Craig A., M.D. "Clostridium Difficile Colitis," eMedicine, Accessed March 9, 2005.
www.emedicine.com/MED/topics3412.htm

"Herpes Simplex Eye Infections," Steen Hall Eye Institute, 2006.
www.steen-hall.com/hsimplex.html

Johnson, Linda A. "Super Bugs' Infect the Super Healthy," *The (Tacoma, Washington) News Tribune*, September 30, 2001.

"Staph Infections Can Be More Than Skin-Deep," *Seattle Post-Intelligencer*, August 17, 2006.

"Study Shows Link Between Antibiotics and Allergies," ScienceDaily, October 1, 2003.
www.sciencedaily.com/releases/2003/10/031001064200.htm

Yee, Daniel. "CDC Recommends New Antibiotics for Gonorrhea," *The Denver Post*, April 13, 2007.

Chapter 14: Chronic Inflammation

Inflammation is a condition that can happen as an acute problem or one that is long term. When inflammation becomes chronic, then the underlying cause must be addressed or it will persist. Localized inflammation should be looked at differently than a chronic systemic problem. Chronic inflammation has been getting more attention in the news lately, due to some recently published studies and books. In several studies dating back to 1998, Harvard University completed studies that pointed to inflammation as being a key factor in the development of high cholesterol and various coronary conditions (Cromie, 1998). More research is pointing to other diseases that seem to have a direct connection to high inflammation in the body (Harvard Health Publications, 2007). Heart disease, strokes, arteriosclerosis (arterial plaque), high blood pressure, diabetes and Alzheimer's are being looked at in a totally different way. Has modern medicine been in the dark ages in its understanding of these conditions and unable to successfully treat these common chronic problems?

I disagree with part of the reasoning from these important studies because it would be impossible for inflammation to actually be the cause of these conditions. Inflammation is nothing more than an effect. Inflammation is the bullet that does the damage, but you must have a gun and a shooter for the bullet to be fired. When you stub your toe, it swells, becomes red, sore and inflamed. Which came first, the toe stub or the inflammation? The heat, swelling and redness, which is the definition of inflammation, is an effect of the injury. Arthritis simply means inflammation of a joint. Colitis means inflammation of the colon. Sinusitis means inflammation of the sinus cavities. Therefore, just as we know that your toe stub created an acute inflammatory state, it is easy to understand that chronic inflammation has to have a cause as well. This does not happen by accident. If you have chronic inflammation in your elbow, for instance, and have never had a serious injury to it, then something has to be causing it. The pain, swelling and redness are an effect of this cause. At some point, if you go to enough health experts, someone will label it as some kind of tendonitis, arthritis, bursitis, etc. Does that tell us what has caused the inflammation, or are the effects of the cause placed in a certain category so we can identify it as a so-called disease?

Systemic Inflammation

When the body is in a state of chronic inflammation, which can be measured by a medical test called C-reactive proteins, is the inflammation the cause or the effect of a bigger pattern? It must be an effect, as something has to cause it. Any "itis" has to have a cause. Looking at possible causes of these "itises" is another way of looking at causes of inflammation. It is one and the same thing.

Chinese medicine points to too much liver heat that comes from a poor diet. This means too much warming food is being consumed, such as greasy and spicy foods, as well as too much alcohol. These foods heat up the liver if consumed regularly. The other causes could include a weak spleen and/or kidneys that may cause the body to not cool properly. This is like a plugged radiator, as the kidney and spleen organs transport fluids. Liver stagnation also creates heat. Too much processed and acid forming foods can also contribute. High insulin spikes have been shown to increase inflammation. Anger and rage also affect the liver by increasing heat. However, many people who have chronic inflammatory patterns eat well and are not angry people. I think the food and emotional imbalances can be more a contributor than a cause. If inflammation already exists, then these foods are feeding the fire.

Rheumatoid arthritis is usually caused by the immune system attacking its own joints, which causes localized inflammation. These attacks and their chemical mediators all contribute to the inflammation. The immune system is very intelligent and is trying to get rid of something, but keeps failing in its attempts. It is trying to get rid of a pathogen or something that is foreign to the body such as a heavy metal substance. I have found that lingering pathogens are the most common denominator in these attacks. These bugs have developed themselves, or evolved enough, to be able to dodge the full onslaught of our immune attacks. They survive and cause havoc. When these attacks become systemic, then we can develop systemic inflammation. The bottom line is that when you have lingering pathogens, you will probably develop some type of either localized and/or systemic inflammation that, if it persists, will cause long-term damage, especially to delicate or previously damaged tissues.

Tissue repair varies depending upon the type of tissue damaged. For instance, working with long-term arthritis patients can be difficult because joint cartilage is slow to repair. More sensitive tissues such as heart valves, eye, lung and nerve tissue may never repair. Stopping the progression of the disease is first and foremost, allowing the patient to make some improvement. However, the healing can be limited by the extent of the damage and its ability to regenerate. Fibromyalgia patients tend to recover much quicker, as muscle tissue is much stronger and tends to hold its own under the inflammatory process.

Allergies

Allergies can also create inflammation. The immune system sees an allergen much like it does a pathogen. Inflammation is created as the body is reacting to a particular substance. That is why an allergy such as dust can create mucus in the sinuses. The mucus is trying to protect the sinuses from the inflammatory process damaging its sensitive lining. If this persists, we have a disease called sinusitis. An allergy to corn sugar, for instance, may cause inflammation in the lungs that can cause an asthma attack or one of several other so-called compartmental lung diseases. Intestinal cramping may be a long-term problem for some that may be due to eating a common food such as wheat. Because it is eaten on a regular basis, you may not get a short-term reaction, but more of a long-term chronic inflammation and stagnation pattern that persists in your intestines. Constipation is an effect of too much heat in the intestines. Too much heat creates the inflammation. Inflammation is usually due to lingering pathogens in the intestines, but can also be a chronic allergic reaction, as I have mentioned.

Pathogens, heavy metals and chronic allergies

Inflammation is the bullet, as it does the damage. The lingering pathogens, heavy metals and chronic allergies are firing the gun. When the body is able to get rid of the pathogens, allergies and heavy metals, the immune system attacks are halted and pain and inflammation are decreased and/or eliminated so normal immune function can return. The body is complex, but exact in its purpose.

Autoimmune/chronic inflammatory conditions happen for a reason. The body is doing what it is supposed to be doing, as it is trying to bring homeostasis to its internal environment. The amount of lingering pathogens, allergies, heavy metals and other foreign substances that are present internally will have a direct correlation to the amount of local or systemic inflammation that coexists in most cases.

Notes

"C-Reactive Protein Test to Screen for Heart Disease: Why Do We Need Another Test?" Harvard Health Publications, Harvard Medical School, Accessed June 7, 2007.
www.health.harvard.edu/newsweek/C-Reactive_Protein_test_to_screen_for_heart_disease.htm

Cromie, William J. "Inflammation May Forecast Heart Attacks," Harvard University Gazette, February 12, 1998.
www.hno.harvard.edu/gazette/1998/02.12/InflammationMay.html

References

Bowman, Lee. "Blood Test Can Predict a Cardiovascular Event," *Seattle Post-Intelligencer*, January 10, 2007.

Cromie, William J. "Better Way to Predict Heart Attacks Is Discovered," Harvard University Gazette, March 23, 2000.
www.hno.harvard.edu/gazette/2000/03.23/heart.html

Dvonch, Louis, M.D., and Russell Dvonch. *The Heart Attack Germ: Prevent Strokes, Heart Attacks, and the Symptoms of Alzheimer's by Protecting Yourself From the Infections and Inflammation of Cardiovascular Disease*. New York: Writer's Showcase, 2003.

Fleming, Richard M., M.D., and Tom Monte. *Stop Inflammation Now!* New York: G.P. Putnam's Sons, 2004.

Liebman, Bonnie. "CRP: Another Piece of the Heart-Disease Puzzle?" *Nutrition Action Healthletter*, March 2003.

Chapter 15: Leaky Gut Syndrome

Leaky gut syndrome is a term that has been used in the alternative medical community for years. Leaky gut is caused by long-term damage to the gut lining, which inhibits the proper assimilation of nutrients. It also causes undigested protein particles and toxics to slip through its damaged lining and enter the bloodstream. The immune system will see these particles as foreign bodies and start attacking them causing an autoimmune type reaction.

The role of pathogens

Pathogenic organisms such as parasites, bacteria and *Candida albicans* overgrowth that have helped to create a chronic inflammatory environment usually do the damage. These organisms set up their residence, usually in the small intestines where the food source is the freshest. *Candida albicans* or yeast overgrowth has been strongly implicated in leaky gut syndrome. This comes from taking antibiotics, birth control pills and steroids. However, any lingering bug will damage the mucosal lining over time. *Candida* and other bugs will burrow themselves into the mucosal lining creating a home in which to multiply and feed off of their favorite host, you. Your intestines are then unable to fully absorb much of your nutrients, and the bugs end up feasting on your food and multiplying at your expense. I also believe that this damaged mucosal environment will also allow some of these foreign invaders to enter into the bloodstream, or the super highway, and end up anywhere they decide best suits their needs.

Allergies

Other inflammatory causes can be from long-term allergic reactions to certain commonly eaten foods, such as wheat, gluten or dairy foods. Since gluten is in so many grains, this irritant can cause chronic inflammation in the gut. This inflammation can be at a low-grade level so that pain may not be present. This type of low-grade inflammation over time can cause permanent damage and intestinal permeability.

Effective gut repair

Many people are given various supplements to help heal the gut wall. This can be helpful. However, as long as the gut is a host for unwanted guests and chronic allergies then healing can only be short lived as the damage continues. The pathogens and allergies must be eliminated before long-term healing can take place. Once they are eliminated, specific nutrition can be added which helps to rebuild and repair the damaged intestinal lining. A quality acidophilus can help, but in addition to this you can add glutamine. This is an amino acid that helps heal the lining. It is one of the best substances for the gut lining repair process as it helps to regenerate healthy tissue. Aloe vera is also effective for repair and helping with gut inflammation. I use several formulas in my practice that combine synergistic ingredients to give maximum repair to the mucosal lining.

See www.richbrightheart.com for information about these products.

References

Kroeger, Hanna. *Parasites, the Enemy Within*, Hanna Kroeger Publications, 1991.

Snyder Sachs, Jessica. "Are Antibiotics Killing Us?" *Discover*, November 2005.

Stein, Rob. "Mystery Intestinal Bug Striking More Patients," *The Olympian*, December 31, 2005.

Chapter 16: Lingering Pathogens

A pathogen is a microorganism that has entered the body, and is capable of producing a disease process. The most familiar pathogens are parasites, viruses and bacteria. Everyone has had a cold or sore throat at some point in their life. These acute symptoms usually arise as a result of a virus or bacteria. Strep throat is from bacteria called *Streptococcus*. A common cold virus, for instance, could be a coronavirus that causes malaise and sinus congestion. Parasites typically cause intestinal problems such as loose stools and cramping. Other less known pathogens are the spirochete *Borrelia burgdorferi* that is transmitted to the body by a tick such as in Lyme disease, mycoplasmas, mycobacteria, and fungal, mold or yeast types such as *Candida albicans*. The difference between an acute pathogen and a lingering one has to do with how long it stays in a person's internal environment.

Pathogens and disease

Hulda Clarke, Ph.D., N.D., wrote a book in 1995 entitled, *The Cure for All Diseases*. She implicated parasites and bacteria as causing many of the so-called diseases of our time, including cancer. I read the book when it was first published and said to myself, "I don't think so." This was a controversial book for its time, and I questioned many aspects of it. I did not dismiss the concept, as it was interesting. I later realized that Hulda Clarke was quite an expert in this field. The only thing I disagree with now, after rereading the book, is that it is not just parasites and bacteria that are doing what she indicated. There are a host of other bugs, some even more destructive to the human body. For that time, she was advanced and right on in her thinking and a pioneer in this area.

While I was in acupuncture school, I had a well-respected and experienced acupuncturist and lecturer for several classes. She spoke often about how lingering pathogens were causing much of the chronic illness of our time. Her way of treating it was to perform acupuncture treatments for thirty consecutive days. I did not think many patients would cooperate with such a protocol, and the acupuncturist needs a few days off as well. However, this stuck in my mind as I suspected some of my patients that were not improving much with the allergy repatterning could have these lingering pathogens underlying their illness. Traditional Chinese Medicine does recognize both acute and lingering pathogens as causative factors in both acute and chronic diseases. Chinese medicine understands that a lingering pathogen can invade the interior of the body and stay there.

During my years in acupuncture training, I had the opportunity to study sixty hours of Toya Hari, which is a form of Japanese acupuncture. They call lingering pathogens the evil qi, which has invaded the interior. I have heard several of my patients tell me that their illness feels like there is something evil living in their body that is constantly attacking them. Evil qi is a good explanation from a Japanese medical perspective, since everything revolves around qi.

The role of the immune system

A normal reaction to a pathogen is that the immune system attacks the pathogen as it enters the system and is able to defeat it. The acute symptoms disappear once the pathogen is removed by the immune system. A lingering pathogen may be too strong for the immune system to overcome, so it survives longer and at some point coexists within the body. It has found a home and is setting up shop. The type and amount of these bugs, the functioning of a person's immune system, and the amount of other internal or external stress determine to what degree these pests grow in numbers and travel to other sites to make a new home.

Some people can live a relatively normal life with a few of these pests coexisting, while other people's health seems to gradually deteriorate as the progression takes place. Pathogens also affect the functioning, directly and indirectly, of organs. They can invade organ tissue and cause a chronic inflammatory pattern that disrupts organ function. The waste products from the pathogens and the subsequent immune attacks put a strain on the liver, spleen and kidneys, which are the eliminative organs. Long-term stress to these organs has cascading effects systemically. As the key eliminative organs wear down, the body's inherent energy systems become depleted. The person's energy level starts to decline and a long-term fatigue pattern sets in. Many people do not realize that there are major internal problems until they hit their forties, as the effects of these bugs are at a symptomatic level. The progression is so slow that many believe that they are just getting older, and it is natural to slow down and have daily pain. They have forgotten what it was like to feel normal.

Symptoms from lingering pathogens

The symptoms from lingering pathogens can vary depending on where the pathogen(s) reside. Many times a chronic sinus infection is a common bacterium called *Staphylococcus aureus*. A form of this particular bacterium is now considered a super bug and is immune to antibiotics. This means that no matter what the antibiotic is that people are taking, the bug will continue to exist within their sinuses and they will continue to have sinusitis, which is inflammation of the sinuses. In fact, the antibiotics have actually made the bacterium stronger, as it has mutated and changed its structural characteristics to survive the antibiotic arsenals that are cast its way. Many epidemiologists are now beginning to recognize this problem and are worried about the future as we have relied so heavily on antibiotic therapy for years. We have overused antibiotics and that is creating these hybrid super bugs. Chapter 19 on Cell Wall Deficient Pathogens gives a full explanation of how physiologically this mutation occurs.

This is an example of just one bug. There are literally hundreds of bugs that can, and do, become lingering pathogens.

Types of pathogens

Various types of pathogens impact the body. Bacteria and viruses are highly active in sinus and respiratory conditions. Bacteria and parasites cause much of the intestinal disorders. Viruses can cause short-term symptoms such as the common cold. But one virus in particular, Epstein-Barr virus, can cause a condition called chronic fatigue syndrome that can be long term. Viruses can also cause mononucleosis as well. Mycoplasmas are major contributors to chronic pain in the body, but can also cause considerable fatigue as well. *Mycoplasma fermentans* was implicated in Gulf War syndrome as many soldiers who came back had symptoms of fibromyalgia, arthritis and chronic fatigue. Many of these soldiers tested positively for this mycoplasma (Nicolson, March 25, 2000).

A mycoplasma has no defined cell wall and can either go unnoticed, or avoid the immune system's attacks since the white blood cells cannot lock onto it in order to destroy it. In fact, it uses other cells, including white blood cells, as hosts. It enters these cells and feeds on their nutrients to nurture its own growth. Many of the so-called autoimmune conditions that are common today are a result of this particular bug. Many of the spouses and children of the soldiers in the Gulf War have now acquired the same germ with similar symptoms. Read Chapter 21 on Mycoplasmas to see how destructive these bugs are.

Ticks can transmit a spirochete that causes Lyme disease, which can result in pain and numbness as well as mental/neurological distress (Fletcher, May 2001). A spirochete is a slender, nonflagellated microorganism. It can enter the spinal cord, meninges (spinal cord membranes), brain and nerve tissue causing much damage. The damage may not be a quick strike, but more a gradual weakening and destruction of tissue. Destruction of nerve tissue causes both pain and/or numbness. Ticks may not kill a person, but may make life miserable, and eventually may cause paralysis.

Pathogens in the body

What happens when a common parasite such as *Blastocystis hominis* enters the digestive tract following the ingestion of water? The parasite begins to grow in numbers and in strength. It will initially cause loose stools and intestinal cramping as the body tries to get rid of it. Parasites will initially set up shop in the small intestine; this is where the feeding is best. Eventually they can enter the spinal cord and even the brain. However, the intestines are the long-term home that they prefer since the food source is most plentiful. As they set up shop, the immune system is trying to frantically seek out and destroy them, much like what happens in the sinuses. Sometimes the immune system is successful, but many times it cannot overcome the type and amount of invaders that are present. We now have a new bug that is coexisting within the intestines and will not leave.

Symptoms, such as intestinal pain and cramping, alternating loose stools and/or constipation, become long-term conditions, just like the chronic sinus infection. Eventually this may turn into chronic constipation as the dominant symptom. Constipation is an effect from too much heat in the intestines. The heat dries up everything including the stool. This could eventually turn into irritable bowel syndrome, Crohn's disease or colitis. These diagnoses made by traditional medical doctors generally mean there is an irritation or inflammation within the digestive system. They do not know the cause, but have categorized symptoms and effects, and have called it a disease. Inflammation is the key word here as any "itis," such as colitis, arthritis, diverticulitis, sinusitis, vaginitis, etc., all refer to an inflammatory pattern somewhere in the body. Doctors do recognize that sinusitis, vaginitis and bladder infections can be caused by a bacterium or *Candida albicans*. Then why is it such a stretch to even begin to understand that other "itises," such as the ones above, can be from the same source? How can a person have inflammation in the sinuses caused by a bacterium, but not the same bug or a different one in the shoulder causing inflammation? The body is a unit that is connected by many types of links, not segmented pieces. These connective pathways include the blood, nerve and lymph systems, as well as the Chinese meridian system. Remember when it was discovered that ulcers were caused by the bacterium *Helicobacter pylori*? Traditional medicine thought it was a lifestyle disease for years. Tuberculosis was also thought to be a lifestyle disease as well, and later it was discovered to be a mycobacterium. I had a young male patient whom I spoke to on the phone tell me that he has had twenty-two surgeries for an aggressive staph infection acquired in the hospital that would not go away. They wanted to amputate his leg. These are all considered lingering pathogens.

How are these bugs acquired? Many people are born with them. Others acquire them through sexual intercourse, on airplanes and from enclosed office buildings, ingestion of food and water, and mosquito bites. See Chapter 18: Acquiring Pathogens.

Inflammation from pathogens

This is a simple concept to grasp. Inflammation is created by two things; first, the presence of a pathogen and second, the constant assault of the immune system trying to seek out and destroy it. When these attacks go on long term, then a chronic inflammatory pattern exists. This can get bad enough that systemic inflammation sets in, which has other repercussions. Any medical doctor or nurse who has worked in a hospital knows that *Staph*, *Strep* or any other bacteria can go anywhere and cause problems. Knee joints, toes, elbows and even the brain are targets for these invaders. Meningitis means inflammation of the meningeal tissue that surrounds the spinal cord. A virus or bacterium often causes this. It is not that much of a stretch then to understand that many pathogens have the ability to invade healthy tissue anywhere in the body including organs and glands, thereby causing localized inflammation. This localized inflammation can start to cause permanent damage to any tissue. A diseased organ may have a certain bacterium or mycoplasma within it that is causing inflammation and progressive damage. Symptoms of intestinal pain and constipation and the diagnosis of colitis only tell us that there is inflammation in the colon. Taking pain medications, laxatives and restricting the diet does nothing to change the underlying pattern. The diagnosis neither tells us what is causing it, nor how to fix it. It is like taking a car to a mechanic because the engine is getting more sluggish and making loud clunking sounds. The mechanic puts a larger muffler on and says, "We don't know what causes this, but the new muffler will help reduce the noise, and the car is getting older, so that is probably why it is slowing down." Most people would immediately run to another mechanic. Just like a car, the body always has a reason why it is not functioning properly. A drug to treat the symptom in this sense is nothing more than a larger new shiny muffler and has no chance of repairing the actual malfunction. In fact, it allows these problems to fester, which can lead to more serious conditions if left improperly treated. Because of our programming by the medically oriented media, we have accepted "muffler-type" treatments as status quo without stopping to question the rationality of thinking behind the diagnosis and treatment. More people in this country would question their mechanic before challenging their doctor.

I have seen thousands of patients with chronic inflammatory patterns labeled arthritis, colitis, irritable bowel syndrome, fibromyalgia, Crohn's disease, gastroesophageal reflux disease, lupus, multiple sclerosis, bursitis, tendonitis, sinusitis and others. The one consistency throughout this process has been: once the source of the problem, usually a pathogen(s) or toxin(s), is removed by the immune system, or by cleansing, then the pain and inflammation seem to subside in conjunction with the removal process.

Notes

Fletcher, J.D. and Tom Klaber. "Lyme Disease: The Unknown Epidemic," *Alternative Medicine*, May 2001.

Nicolson, Garth L., Ph.D. "VA Confirms Nicholson's Data on Chronic Infections in Gulf War Illness Patients," The Institute for Molecular Medicine, March 25, 2000. www.immed.org/illness/whatsnew/news00-3-25.html

References

Brownstein, David, M.D. *Overcoming Arthritis*. West Bloomfield, Michigan: Medical Alternatives Press, 2001.

"Chlamydia," National Institutes of Health, National Institute of Allergy and Infectious Diseases, August 2006. www.niaid.nih.gov/factsheets/stdclam.htm

Clarke, Hulda, Ph.D., N.D. *The Cure for All Diseases*. Chula Vista, California: New Century Press, 1995.

Deadman, Peter and Mazin Al-Khafaji. *A Manual of Acupuncture*. Vista, California: Eastland Press, 1998.

Dvonch, Louis, M.D., and Russell Dvonch. *The Heart Attack Germ: Prevent Strokes, Heart Attacks, and the Symptoms of Alzheimer's by Protecting Yourself From the Infections and Inflammation of Cardiovascular Disease*. New York: Writer's Showcase, 2003.

Jaret, Peter. "Nano–The Deadly Little Creatures That Could Change the Way You Think About Your Health," *Alternative Medicine*, March 2003.

Johnson, Linda A. "Staph Strain Infects More Healthy People," *Seattle Post-Intelligencer,* September 30, 2004.

Levine, Arnold J. *Viruses.* New York: Scientific American Library, 1992.

Murphy, Kate. "Bacteria's Expanding Reach Elicits Concern," *International Herald Tribune*, August 24, 2006.

Nicolson, Garth L., Ph.D. "Chronic Fatigue Illnesses," The Institute for Molecular Medicine, Accessed June 26, 2005. www.immed.org/illness/infectious_disease_research.html

Nicolson, Garth L., Ph.D. "Chronic Infectious Diseases," The Institute for Molecular Medicine, Accessed June 26, 2005. www.immed.org/illness/fatigue_illness_research.html

Nicolson, Garth L., Ph.D. "Autoimmune Illnesses and Degenerative Diseases," The Institute for Molecular Medicine, Accessed June 26, 2005. www.immed.org/illness/fatigue_autoimmune_illness_research.html

Ojcius, David M., Toni Darville and Patrick M. Bavoil. "Can Chlamydia Be Stopped?" *Scientific American*, May 2005.

Paulson, Tom. "Antibiotics Prompt Bacteria 'Walls," *The Olympian,* August 25, 2005.

Poehlmann, Katherine M., Ph.D. *Rheumatoid Arthritis: The Infection Connection–Targeting and Treating the Cause of Chronic Illness.* Rolling Hills Estates, California: Satori Press, 2002.

"Report Rates of Infections in Hospitals," *The Olympian*, February 2, 2007.

Sinha, Gunjan. "Gulf War Illness: Psychological?" *Popular Science*, April 1999.

Snyder Sachs, Jessica. "Are Antibiotics Killing Us?" *Discover*, November 2005.

"Staph Infections Can Be More Than Skin-Deep," *Seattle Post-Intelligencer*, August 17, 2006.

Tacoma-Pierce County Health Department and Spokane Regional Health Department. "Living with MRSA (Methicillin-Resistant Staphylococcus Aureus)," Fall 2004.

Yee, Daniel. "CDC Recommends New Antibiotics for Gonorrhea," *The Denver Post*, April 13, 2007.

Chapter 17: Inside the Mind of a Pathogen

I would love to get into the mind of a pathogen and see what makes it tick. The only problem is that they do not have a brain, or do they? Just for the fun of it, here is what a conversation with a bacterium might sound like.

"Hi, my name is Mr. Bad Bug, and I'm part of a like-minded group called *Staphylococcus aureus*. Survival at all cost is the name of the game. I need to feed myself in order to survive. I love sugar and hormones the best. Some of the less fortunate bugs have to take over other cells and use their nutrients for survival. We are more evolved than they are. We like to live in certain areas as long as the food supply is adequate. Our gang tends to hang out in the sinuses and ears a lot. It is nice and moist there. When our group gets too large, we have to venture out into uncharted territory for fresh supplies of food and enough space to stretch out and raise a large family. Sometimes we can move just a few streets over, so the capillaries are the route. When we get tired of hanging out in the sinuses, we may want to take an extended vacation and go somewhere exotic. We may want to travel to an area that is less populated, so we can kick back and relax. We'll take the super highway that you guys call an artery. Then we'll take the expressway, or as you call them, the arterioles, and find the right capillary exit and head straight for the knee joint. I hear there's a wonderful food supply there as joints get fresh blood daily.

"Some of the other bugs, such as parasites, bacteria and *Candida,* prefer the intestinal tract. There's always a supply of fresh food in there, so they can feast on it often. Those *Candida* bugs just love their sugar, bread and cheeses. Spirochetes transmitted by ticks prefer the nervous system, brain and spinal cord. My friends, the mycoplasmas, love joints, organs, muscles and taking over other cells. *Chlamydia pneumoniae* love the lungs, heart and coronary arteries. My cousin, *Streptococcus*, usually hangs out in the throat and lungs. Myself, I prefer the ear and sinuses, as it's very cozy in there. I don't know why certain bug populations prefer some areas to others. They just seem to adapt better to certain environments. But, aren't you humans much the same way?

"You keep throwing those antibiotics at us. At one time, they threw us for a loop, but we have evolved and mutated into stronger forms in order to survive. We can even change our appearance by changing our exterior cell walls in order to evade those pesky white blood cells. Many times we go hide out in certain areas so the antibiotics can't get to us. Some of us are even stealth-like so we can change forms in order to squeeze in and out of narrow places. We can hide in places that once were impossible to gain access to. We can even hide out in your very own lymphocytes, those white blood cells that accumulate when there's chronic injury or irritation, to avoid detection. Some of us have even developed a film-like material that we produce in order to surround us and protect us from the antibiotics and immune attacks. I hear the nanobacteria produce a calcium shell so your immune system can't even detect them.

"I don't know if you humans realize it, but we're winning this war. You keep sending new types of antibiotics after us, but we're way too strong now. This is getting far too easy. Hopefully you humans don't come up with any new weapons that can stop our progress."

Chapter 18: Acquiring Pathogens

Many people ask me, "How in the world did I get bugs?" There is a lack information or misinformation on the types of pathogens and how they find their way into our domain.

The birth process

Much of this pathogenic sharing starts in the uterus before birth. Mom has a bug that is transferred to the fetus while it is forming. At what point the bug enters is unknown. Through the umbilical cord we receive all the nutrients we need to begin the life process. We also get some things that may be to our detriment as well. Dad may also pass the bug on during the ejaculation process by releasing a pathogen into the vaginal tract. From there it can find its way into the egg. Remember, it is not a single bug that is the problem, but perhaps thousands of a single variety or multiple varieties that can infect an area or body part.

Many babies that are born with birth defects such as mental retardation or brain damage and are born premature and/or stillborn are victims of infection within the womb. Many times a baby born sickly is a reflection of this problem. There are times when pathogenic entry happens during delivery, no matter how sterile the environment is. Many hospital nurses and delivery room specialists carry *Staphylococcus aureus*, as well as other pathogens. Therefore, it is impossible to ensure noncontamination during the birth process. We know that the parasite *Toxoplasma gondii* is readily passed on to the fetus during pregnancy. A recent report stated that hospitals feared up to 40 percent of expecting mothers may carry this parasite. This bug is commonly acquired from cat litter boxes, as it can be inhaled. This parasite is one of the leading causes of brain damage, and has only recently come to our awareness. All expecting mothers should be tested for it.

Your partner

The second and most common way to share pathogens is with your partner. We have all been schooled regarding gonorrhea, chlamydia, herpes simplex 1 and 2 and AIDS. We can be tested for them prior to a new relationship, so we can feel better about sharing body fluids. This is important; however, there may be a much bigger picture potentially brewing. You may have a partner that is the model of health, but may be a carrier for any type of bug. That bug may have been held in check for years by your partner strong immune system. You can be the recipient of such a gift at any point of contact.

Transference of pathogens is much easier if you have a partner that has multiple pathogens within his/her system and his/her health is suspect. Transference depends on many factors: the strength of your immune system, the type of bugs your partner is carrying, the strength in numbers of the pathogens, and the location within your partner's body. For example, if you have a partner who has a chronic sinus infection and *Staphylococcus aureus* is the culprit, then your chance of getting *Staphylococcus aureus* from your partner is high with open-mouth kissing. This is because *Staphylococcus aureus* is living in your partner's sinuses and those mucus membranes are adjacent to the mouth. This is a relatively easy transference. Your immune system may ward it off for a while. However, at any point you may not be able to hold it back, and you start to develop a symptom in the head that is not characteristic of your prior history. You may get a headache, earache, eye infection or stuffy nose that will not go away because you are getting repeated doses every time you kiss your partner.

Streptococcus is another common bacterium that can be shared by kissing. The throat is the basement floor of the mouth. Both *Staphylococcus* and *Streptococcus* become part of your saliva when exchanged on a regular basis with a partner. Other bacteria, some common cold viruses and mycobacterium can be shared, as well, by kissing. Cytomegalovirus is referred to as the kissing virus.

The sex organs

The next mode of entry is through sexual organs. Besides the bugs mentioned above we have a host of opportunists just waiting for a chance to get in for an extended stay. We know about the commonly named sexual bugs. But lesser known ones can potentially cause long-term suffering for you and your partner. *Urea ureaplasma, Trichomonas vaginalis, Mycoplasma hominis, Candida albicans, Gardnerella vaginalis, Mycoplasma genitalium, Mycoplasma fermentans, Mycoplasma penetrans* and human papillomavirus (HPV or wart virus), especially HPV 15 and HPV 16, are some of the common pathogens that can gain entry. Again, entrance is easy with intercourse, especially passing from male to female. Anything that is being carried by either partner in the genital area, urinary tract and/or bloodstream has a high risk for transmission. I think that much prostatitis, prostate cancer, vaginitis, vaginal cysts, tumors, cervical cancer, cervical dysplasia, fallopian tube disorders, pelvic inflammatory disease and other diseases can potentially have their roots in sharing pathogens during sexual intercourse. As proof of this, a drug company recently introduced a vaccine for HPV, which is indicated in cervical cancer.

Unfortunately, even after being tested and given a clean bill of sexual health does little to guarantee that these other bugs cannot be potential contaminants. Many of these bugs are out of the radar of normal testing procedures due to either a lack of awareness of their potential to cause illness, or to the lack of the ability to accurately test individuals. The expense and timeframe for some of this testing is another factor as cultures may need lengthy periods to reveal certain pathogenic strains. We only recently have been able to devise tests that can detect mycoplasma infection. Mycoplasmas have only been recognized as being pathogenic in the last decade. Still most health care providers are completely unaware of their potential for disease, let alone their existence. All people should be tested for mycoplasma infection, as well as all the above bugs, including Lyme disease. The Gulf War was proof that many of the partners of those infected and their children became eventually positive themselves for mycoplasma infection.

Good hygiene and protection

Therefore, it is prudent to be aware that increased sexual partners and unprotected sexual intercourse sets you up for potential pathogenic entry. You may be in a secure long-term relationship with a seemingly healthy partner who appears safe on the surface but may have the potential for illness to arise, as one of you may be a carrier for a certain pathogenic strain. The best thing to do is be aware and use good hygiene and protection. Inspect your groin area on a regular basis for any possible sign of rashes, bumps or discharge, especially if one of these presents itself following intercourse. Becoming ill within the first year or two after starting a sexual relationship may have something to do with specific pathogens that your partner is sharing with you.

References

Hamza, Haizal, M.D. "Bacterial Infections and Pregnancy," eMedicine, Accessed June 8, 2005.
www.emedicine.com/med/topic3269.htm

Keane, Sandy. "Mycoplasma and Miscarriage," *Maternal Health News,* Vol. 10, No. 2, n.d.

Nicolson, Garth L., Ph.D. "Chronic Infectious Diseases," The Institute for Molecular Medicine, Accessed June 26, 2005.
www.immed.org/illness/fatigue_illness_research.html

Ojcius, David M., Toni Darville and Patrick M. Bavoil. "Can Chlamydia Be Stopped?" *Scientific American*, May 2005.

Chapter 19: Cell Wall Deficient Pathogens

The ability of the body to form structures to serve its function is fascinating. The basic concept is that structure always determines function, especially at a microscopic level.

Cell wall deficient pathogens are actually becoming very common and are responsible for much of the chronic illness we see today. These pathogens have altered cell walls, which give them characteristics that are different from a normal bacterium. They may be a subculture of a classic bacteria or fungi which has changed form. They are also referred to as L-forms. Their growth requirement may be altered, and they may have colonies that are not typical of their parent cells. Some of these cells actually flourish inside both red and white blood cells and tissue cells. They can invade these cells due to their microscopic size, cell wall alterations and ability to change shapes. They are sometimes referred to as stealth pathogens or pleomorphic types.

Cell wall changes

Cell wall deficient (CWD) means the cell wall has been altered. This usually takes place in response to the presence of antibiotic therapy. The change in structure of the cell wall is due to its ability to alter itself for pure survival in the presence of antibiotics. A bacterium such as *Staphylococcus aureus* will become a CWD or L-form. The main change occurs in the cell wall due to its loss of rigidity. This wall has within it a murein layer that consists of glucosamine, thamnose and muramic acid. The lack of muramic acid is a change that takes place that contributes to this loss of rigidity. In addition, it builds a substitute polysaccharide wall of glucose, galactose and rhamnose. The lipid component in the wall is increased up to four times in some species. The protein peptide density is lessened. The overall density of the membrane goes from a high molecular weight to low. The other component change will be the addition of diaminopimelic acid (DAP). DAP is a component of this plastic wall. Its function is to prevent the wall from reforming and becoming more rigid. This, however, is not a set pattern for all CWD pathogen cell wall alterations. There can be variances within the new design, which accommodate that particular pathogenic species. The main thing to understand is that this is an example of how genetic mutation and adaptation take place in any species. The cell wall becomes less dense, or loosely integrated. The cell has the ability to change shapes more readily and function as an almost distinct entity from the parent form. It also has the ability to survive the changing environment of antibiotic warfare. This is not any different from any animal or plant species that evolve in order to survive (Mattman, 2001).

The impact on organs

CWD pathogens target organs more readily than their parent species. When a CWD or L-form of a bacterium invades countless red blood cells, the immune system sees its own blood as a foreign entity. It can become very confused. Those red blood cells also lose their ability to function, which leads to blood deficiency or anemic problems. No wonder there are so many sick people with various autoimmune illnesses. When your own blood becomes a foreign entity to your immune system and goes under attack, then this is truly the definition of an autoimmune disease. Almost every species of bacteria has L-forms within its species once it is exposed to antibiotics. This variant strain is its survival mechanism. When a species becomes densely populated, it has the ability to survive more readily under attack.

Penicillin seems to be the antibiotic that induces the most changes in cell wall mutations. With *Candida albicans*, the antifungal drug nystatin produces similar results with this yeast or fungus type. Nanobacteria build a calcium shell around themselves in order to avoid the immune and antibiotic attacks. Calcium, being a natural component of the body, is bypassed by the immune system. This is why cell wall deficient pathogens are so dangerous. They can disguise themselves as something other than what they are. Mycoplasmas are born cell wall deficient. They are the most dangerous pathogenic entity next to the AIDS virus (Mattman, 2001).

CWD pathogens are the root of what is causing so much chronic illness in our country. These pathogens, such as mycoplasmas, cell wall altered types of bacteria and mycobacteria, are creating a devastating impact on our health. So much illness today is due to these well-developed pathogens. The sad thing is that very few health care professionals even know they exist. I talk with many intelligent alternative doctors and other health care professionals and am amazed at the lack of awareness. This knowledge needs to be taught at all traditional and nontraditional medical schools. We are still in the dark ages when it comes to this much-needed understanding.

Lida Mattman's book, *Cell Wall Deficient Forms–Stealth Pathogens*, offers scientific proof of the existence of CWD pathogens and how they function.

Notes

Mattman, Lida H. *Cell Wall Deficient Forms–Stealth Pathogens*. Boca Raton, Florida: CRC Press LLC, 2001.

References

Johnson, Linda A. "Super Bugs' Infect the Super Healthy," *The (Tacoma, Washington) News Tribune*, September 30, 2001.

"Rheumatoid Arthritis and Multiple Sclerosis–The Cause May Be in the Blood," *Alternative Medicine Digest*, Issue No. 18, 1996.

Tacoma-Pierce County Health Department and Spokane Regional Health Department. "Living with MRSA (Methicillin-Resistant Staphylococcus Aureus)," Fall 2004.

Jaret, Peter. "Nano–The Deadly Little Creatures That Could Change the Way You Think About Your Health," *Alternative Medicine*, March 2003.

Chapter 20: Mycobacteria

Researchers are becoming more aware of the impact that mycobacteria can have on chronic health conditions. These subcultures of bacteria are very slow moving. They have both fungal and bacterial characteristics. They belong to the broader family called Actinomycetes. They include *Nocardia, Corynebacterium, Mycobacterium avium intracellulare, Mycobacterium avium complex* and *Mycobacterium tuberculosis* (tuberculosis bacteria). These mycobacteria can also become cell wall deficient (CWD) or L-form, as a subcolony of the parent, and can revert back to the parent form as well. (See Chapter 19: Cell Wall Deficient Pathogens.) *Nocardia* is very close in its structure to *Mycobacterium tuberculosis*. It also resembles the bacterium *Listeria* that has been implicated in certain types of cancer, arthritis and scleroderma.

Nocardia and Parkinson's

In 1994, researchers B. Beaman and B.L. Beaman inoculated mice with *Nocardia*. The mice developed movement and behavioral problems, which are similar to Parkinson's disease. Another study in 1991 by two Japanese microbiologists, S. Kohbata and K. Shimokawa at the Gifu School of Medicine, showed positive antibodies for *Nocardia* in twenty out of twenty patients who had Parkinson's. The base of the brain is the area that houses the dopamine receptors. This area includes the substantia nigra, the basal ganglia and the proximal cranial nerves. These cranial nerves control facial expression, among other things. This area becomes inflamed and turns fibrous much like any area of the body that has chronic inflammation. The deterioration of the substantia nigra and its neurons is considered the primary cause in Parkinson's. This is where the dopamine receptors are located. A depletion of the neurotransmitter dopamine occurs. The damage also impacts the adjacent cranial nerves, which affect facial expression (Broxmeyer, 2002).

Researchers suspect that it may not be the rod-shaped *Nocardia* that is actually doing the damage. However, they think the damage is caused by the round-shaped L-form, or CWD form of *Nocardia* that is entering into this delicate area. The less rigid shape and microscopic size of the L-form *Nocardia* is able to pass through the blood-brain barrier and settle itself into the base of the brain. Central nervous system tuberculosis has symptoms that seem to mimic Parkinson's. *Nocardia* may just be a variant strain of the *Mycobacterium tuberculosis*.

Other mycobacteria

Corynebacterium diphtheriae is another mycobacterium that causes heart, lung, kidney and peripheral nerve disorders. It usually enters the system through the lungs, genitalia or eyes. It produces a toxin that causes damage to the above areas. *Mycobacterium avium intracellulare* has been implicated in lung disorders in immune compromised individuals.

I recently worked with an eight-year-old girl who was losing her eyesight. It was deteriorating rapidly. I suspected that one or more mycobacterium may be at the root of this. Following several treatment sessions, her eyesight quickly returned to normal. Since then she has been fine. I believe this happened because those mycobacteria were sitting in the area of the brain that affects the optic nerve. These mycobacteria caused localized inflammation and damage to this nerve, which lead to the deterioration of her eyesight.

Mycobacteria as causative agents

Any of these pathogens can cause disease. They are slow moving, so illness can present itself over decades. Because of their size and varying shapes, mycobacteria should be looked at as primary causative agents in various diseases, as well as other cerebral meningeal/spinal disorders. They have the ability to enter areas that normal bacteria and viruses cannot invade due to their shape, size and altered cell wall structure. Once entrenched, they can cause a long-term, low-grade inflammatory process (Broxmeyer, 2002 and Mattman, 2001).

The basic premise is that if an area such as the substantia nigra in Parkinson's patients is deteriorating, then something has to be causing it. This information seems the most plausible for a causative agent. I believe that possibly other cell wall deficient pathogenic species, including mycoplasmas, parasites, spirochetes and variant strains of bacteria, as well as heavy metals and toxins also have the ability to cause Parkinson's disease, in addition to a host of other illnesses, which seem to have no known cause.

Notes

Broxmeyer, Lawrence, M.D. *Parkinson's–Another Look*. Chula Vista, California: New Century Press, 2002.

Mattman, Lida H. *Cell Wall Deficient Forms–Stealth Pathogens*. Boca Raton, Florida: CRC Press LLC, 2001.

Chapter 21: Mycoplasmas

Mycoplasmas are the smallest self-replicating pathogens known to man. They are considered pleomorphic or stealth-like because of their unstable characteristics and amazing ability to change shape and structure instantaneously.

The role of mycoplasmas

Mycoplasmas are simple forms of bacteria; however, they are not true bacteria as they cannot synthesize nutrients. Mycoplasmas are just starting to come to the forefront as primary causative agents in many types of the chronic and degenerative diseases of our time. This is mainly due to the recent advances in our ability to accurately detect them in laboratory testing. This discovery is spawning new clinical research.

Mycoplasmas are the tricksters of the immune system. Mycoplasmas are able to rob other cells of their nutrients by invading host cells and using the host cell's lipids and internal components to incorporate into the mycoplasmas' own surface structure. The immune system can be tricked into attacking these once healthy cells, due to their changed cell structure. They can change their surface structure to avoid being attacked, or even disappear if needed. Mycoplasmas can also disguise themselves inside other cells that they use as hosts, so as not to be detected by the immune system. They can even take over and disrupt the functioning of white blood cells. Mycoplasmas can live inside a white blood cell and get a free ride across the blood-brain barrier ending up in the brain, spinal cord or anywhere else they would like to be. They can enter other cells as well, including red blood cells and various tissue structures.

Mycoplasmas can use lipids from the mitochondria of healthy cells, which causes that cell to lose electrons and in turn contributes to cellular fatigue. This is what often causes the fatigue in fibromyalgia and chronic fatigue syndrome. In lab studies, mycoplasmas have shown the ability to infect non-cancerous cells by turning them more malignant. Mycoplasmas can cause plaque to form inside artery walls much like bacteria have been proven to do. They have the ability to stimulate proinflammatory cytokine production. Cytokines are chemicals that call out to other immune system components to come and join the battle, which is a double-edged sword as inflammation is increased as well. We know how damaging chronic inflammation can be to tissue structures such as joints, blood vessels, heart valves and brain and nerve tissue (Guthrie, September 2001).

Mycoplasmas have similar cell wall deficient characteristics that mycobacteria and mutated bacteria possess. The difference is that mycoplasmas are faster acting and much more aggressive. Their membrane is very lucid, having little structure. It is mostly composed of water and fat. This gives mycoplasmas the ability to change shape and surface components at will, easily and quickly, in order to avoid being detected. Mycoplasmas are impossible to detect in culture samples that use conventional lab methods that test for antibodies. They infect other species and plants as well as humans (Mattman, 2001 and Nicolson, June 26, 2005).

Mycoplasmas and serious illnesses

Although not all mycoplasmas are pathogenic to humans, these seven mycoplasmas are responsible for many serious illnesses. They are the most important ones to be aware of.

Public enemy number one is *Mycoplasma fermentans*. This bug is at the top of the most human destructive list. It is directly responsible for, or at least a major contributor to, the majority of autoimmune conditions and chronic fatiguing illnesses that are now epidemic in our society. Many studies have found this bug in the synovial fluids of rheumatoid arthritis sufferers. *Mycoplasma fermentans* is the leading cause of arthritis. It has also been found in the bone marrow of children who have leukemia. This is the most aggressive of all the mycoplasmas in terms of its ability to be resistant and invasive in its attempts to take over the body.

Mycoplasma incognitus is structurally very similar to *mycoplasma fermentans*. However, it acts differently in the body. *Mycoplasma incognitus* loves the brain and spinal cord and is responsible for numerous neurological symptoms, including memory loss, mental confusion, depression, anxiety, Reynaud's disease, spinal pain, headaches and many other symptoms.

The next in line is *Mycoplasma genitalium*. This mycoplasma has been isolated consistently in the genital-urinary system as a primary contributor to pelvic inflammatory disease, urogenital problems and urethritis, as well as respiratory disorders. It also is a major contributor to various chronic and debilitating illnesses including chronic joint pain.

Another dangerous mycoplasma is *Mycoplasma pneumoniae*, which is known to be one of the chief culprits in numerous lung conditions including pneumonia. This bug was the first mycoplasma identified, as well as the most commonly recognized by allopathic medicine as a causative agent in pneumonia. *Mycoplasma pneumoniae* just recently received national attention as a possible cause of chronic asthma.

Also treacherous is *Mycoplasma salivarium*. Once in the bloodstream, it can go anywhere, but it has a tendency to locate in the joints where it causes chronic inflammation.

Next on the most wanted list is *Mycoplasma hominis*. This pest is responsible for much of the pelvic inflammatory disease seen today, and it causes many genital/uterine conditions, as well.

The next popular criminal is *Ureaplasma urealyticum*, which is known to cause urinary tract infections, pelvic inflammatory problems and urethritis, among other things.

The last, but not least, is *Mycoplasma penetrans*. This pathogen is indicated in both joint and muscle problems. I think it may be the primary underlying cause in many cases of fibromyalgia and other soft tissue related chronic inflammatory conditions as well as chronic fatigue syndrome.

There is concern that mycoplasmas play a large role in many types of cancers. For starters, they are immune to our own white blood cells. Secondly, they take over and have the ability to invade without destroying any type of cell in the body. They can use our white blood cells as a host for the nutrients they need. These white blood cells are our defense for preventing illness, including cancer. Third, and most important, they help drive the progression of cancer cells and help to increase their malignant nature by helping to spread these cancer cells throughout the body. They even increase the release of free radicals within the body, thereby causing free radical damage, which is known to cause, or at least contribute to, cancer and other diseases.

Why is so little known about these bugs and so little medical research being done? The Gulf War created more than one hundred thousand soldiers who came back with Gulf War syndrome. Forty percent of these tested positive for mycoplasma infection, and of those, 80 percent showed positive for *Mycoplasma fermentans*. Many of their family members and even their pets have become ill due to this bug. A husband-and-wife team, Garth and Nancy Nicolson, who are well-known researchers, conducted these tests (Nicolson, March 25, 2000). Garth Nicolson, Ph.D., held the chair at the University of Texas in cancer research. His wife Nancy Nicolson was a former instructor at the Baylor College of Medicine in the Department of Immunology and Microbiology. Nancy had suffered herself from mycoplasma infection years earlier. They became involved in their own independent study because their daughter was one of those infected during the Gulf War.

I have known countless people infected with mycoplasmas. No one knows how transmission takes place. I believe mycoplasmas can be transmitted sexually and possibly in close quarters with other infected individuals, as well as the most obvious, womb transmission. I am not surprised when a chronically ill person has one of these bugs residing within them. Mycoplasmas are becoming common in our society, just as common as the huge increase in chronic illness, especially autoimmune diseases and cancers. Gulf War illness is a strong indicator of their virulence and ability to cause severe illness. I know that these patients are usually the sickest ones that I see. When you combine more than one mycoplasma in a body, then the symptoms are exacerbated even more.

Alternative Medicine and *Nexus New Times* magazines ran features on mycoplasma infection. The Internet has a wealth of information on these critters. Their effect in deteriorating immune function alone opens the door for other opportunist pathogens to come on in and crash the party. If people knew the impact in our society that these bugs are having in terms of chronic illness, suffering, medical expense and lost lives, they would be in shock. I believe that at least 50 percent of our population is currently infected by mycoplasmas. This percentage is growing as the spreading of these organisms is on the rise.

How many countless Americans are chronically ill without knowing that these are the culprits underlying their disease process? Mycoplasmas are in a class by themselves. They take a back seat only to the AIDS virus in terms of their potential to cause death. A mycoplasma may not directly kill you as AIDS can, but it may make your life so miserable that it could seem as though dying might be a better option. Everyone in this country should be screened for these bugs, as this silent epidemic has gained much momentum and has entrenched itself deeply into our society.

Notes

Guthrie, Michael, R.PH. "Mycoplasmas: The Missing Link in Fatiguing Illness," *Alternative Medicine*, September 2001.

Mattman, Lida H. *Cell Wall Deficient Forms–Stealth Pathogens.* Boca Raton, Florida: CRC Press LLC, 2001.

Nicolson, Garth L., Ph.D. "Chronic Infectious Diseases," The Institute for Molecular Medicine, Accessed June 26, 2005.
www.immed.org/illness/fatigue_illness_research.html

Nicolson, Garth L., Ph.D. "VA Confirms Nicholson's Data on Chronic Infections in Gulf War Illness Patients," The Institute for Molecular Medicine, March 25, 2000.
www.immed.org/illness/whatsnew/news00-3-25.html

References

Baseman, Joel B. and Joseph G. Tully. "Mycoplasmas: Sophisticated, Reemerging and Burdened by Their Notoriety," Centers for Disease Control and Prevention, February 5, 1997. www.cdc.gov/ncidod/eid/Vol3no1/baseman.htm

"Chameleon-Like Microbes May Be Causing Your Chronic or Autoimmune Disorder," *Members Alert for July 2001*, Health Sciences Institute, Vol. 6, No. 1, July 2001.

Chatterjee, Archana, M.D. "Mycoplasma Infections," eMedicine, Accessed March 4, 2005.
www.emedicine.com/ped/topic1524.htm

Keane, Sandy. "Mycoplasma and Miscarriage," *Maternal Health News,* Vol. 10, No. 2, n.d.

Nicolson, Garth L., Ph.D. "Autoimmune Illnesses and Degenerative Diseases," The Institute for Molecular Medicine, Accessed June 26, 2005.
www.immed.org/illness/fatigue_autoimmune_illness_research.html

Nicolson, Garth L., Ph.D. "Chronic Fatigue Illnesses," The Institute for Molecular Medicine, Accessed June 26, 2005.
www.immed.org/illness/infectious_disease_research.html

Rottem, Shalomo. "Interaction of Mycoplasmas With Host Cells," *Physiological Review,* Vol. 83, No. 2, April 2003.

Scott, Donald W. "Mycoplasma and Neurosystemic Diseases," *Nexus New Times Magazine*, Vol. 8, No. 5, September/October 2001.

Sinha, Gunjan. "Gulf War Illness: Psychological?" *Popular Science*, April 1999.

Waites, Ken. B., M.D. "Mycoplasma Infections," eMedicine, Accessed March 14, 2005.
www.emedicine.com/MED/topic1540.htm

Chapter 22: Fungi

Fungi are slow moving pathogenic forms that can take over the body at any given time. They possess unique qualities such as the ability to act as both a pathogen and an allergen. Fungi produce mycotoxins that stimulate immune cells to react, producing strong allergic reactions. Fungi tend to invade and inhabit damp moist places such as the sinus cavities, groin, ears, eyes, and between the toes, as well as the respiratory, vaginal and intestinal tracts.

The role of fungi

Once fungi enter the bloodstream, they can travel to other possible sites of infestation including the brain, skin, spinal cord, joints and organs, especially the pancreas. Typical symptoms include headaches, fatigue, spaciness, vertigo, eczema, ringing in the ears, vaginitis, sinusitis, diarrhea, depression, irritability and joint pain. Allergic reactions to various fungi and the mycotoxins that they produce can cause a multitude of symptoms. For instance, the fungal toxin called aflatoxin in peanuts can cause severe allergic reactions.

The disorders

Many pathogenic forms of fungi can cause respiratory illness (Kaufmann, 2003). Fungi can play key roles in these conditions. Remember, any pathogen that invades the respiratory system, no matter what the pathogenic form, will compromise breathing capacity. This inhabitation can go on for either short or long periods of time depending upon the length of residence. Key fungi involved in disturbing lung and bronchiole function could include *Histoplasma capsulatum*, *Aspergillus*, *Alternaria*, *Candida albicans*, *Blastomyces dermatitidis* and *Coccidioides immitis*.

Sinusitis, as well as ear and eye infections, has been shown to be caused by *Alternaria*, *Aspergillus*, *Cladosporium*, *Penicillium* and *Candida albicans*. Intestinal infections are commonly caused by *Candida albicans* due to antibiotic overuse.

Many times a fungal infection can occur within the central nervous system, which may not be a full-blown acute occurrence such as seen in acute meningitis (Kaufmann, 2000). However, it is a low-grade, chronic, slow-moving infection that may cause depression, anxiety and brain fog due to the persistent pathogenic presence of fungi within the brain and spinal cord. Fungi can also cause a severe bout of acute meningitis as well. *Candida albicans* and *Cryptococcus* are some of the usual suspects.

Several different forms of *Candida* including *Candida albicans*, *Candida krusei* and *Candida rugosa*, as well as several other fungi, can cause vaginitis, prostatitis and urethritis. These pathogenic forms can be passed back and forth during sexual intercourse. Women who have vaginal yeast infections from *Candida* can transfer this yeast to the male during sexual intercourse. The yeast will back up into the prostate gland causing a low-grade, long-term inflammatory reaction to occur. Other fungi may also be present adding to the dilemma. These bugs are ever present and slow moving so that an illness such as prostatitis can take years to come about.

Candida and other fungi forms, as well as the mycotoxins that they secrete, can cause painful arthritic joint pain (Kaufmann, 2000).

Fungi and the immune system

What fungi generally do is compromise immune function as they enter the blood stream and tissue, creating havoc. A weakened immune system caused by a chronic fungal infection is much more susceptible to other invading microbes. Again, it can be seen how the improper use of antibiotics plays such an important role in compromising immune function by creating an unhealthy systemic environment that places the body in a vulnerable position for further chronic infections. As mentioned above, fungi also can enter the bloodstream and enter the joints causing arthritic type symptoms (Kaufmann, 2000).

Fungal infections need to be looked at more closely so they can be considered as possible candidates for a broad spectrum of both acute and chronic illnesses. Many fungal infections occur because of a weakened immune system. The weakened immune system comes about as a reflection of the pathogenetic imprint that has been left to us by our parents, the overuse of antibiotics and the way we have chosen to live our lives.

Notes

Kaufmann, Doug. *The Fungus Link: An Introduction to Fungal Disease Including the Initial Phase Diet*. Rockwall, Texas: Media Trition Inc., 2000.

Kaufmann, Doug. *The Fungus Link: Volume 2, Tracking the Cause*. Rockwall, Texas: Media Trition Inc., 2003.

Chapter 23: Oxidative Stress

Oxidative stress is a new term that is gaining attention. It is the effect of how reactive oxygen affects the body over time. An oxidative stress test is a way of measuring the amount of reactive oxygen or free radical damage that is occurring inside the body at a cellular level. Free radicals are continually being formed in the body. They are known to cause DNA and cell membrane damage, as well as premature aging. Free radical damage is associated with many degenerative illnesses.

The role of oxidative stress

Oxidative stress and free radical damage increase the likelihood that the body is breaking down at a faster rate than normal. This ongoing damage can be measured as a marker much like C-reactive protein is measured as an inflammation marker. Oxidative stress and inflammation are two key indicators of heart disease, stroke, diabetes and many other chronic deteriorating illnesses including cancer.

Oxidative stress over time changes the way cells function by altering the structure and the function of the cell and its membrane. Signal transduction pathways are sensitive to reactive oxygen (Gottschling, 2001). These pathways transmit key cellular communication from the cell's surface (membrane) into the nucleus. Oxidative stress damages these pathways by deteriorating the cells lipids, proteins and DNA. Because the cell has a lipid bi-layer, damage will occur within this delicate membrane greatly influencing cellular signaling and communication. With a cell's membrane impaired, a lack of nutrient absorption and cellular detoxification occurs. The cell basically shuts down and the disease process ensues. This leads to the initiation and progression of mutational events. Cell mutation is a key determinant in the development of cancerous cells, as well as many other chronic conditions (Gottschling, 2001).

Reactive oxygen species

The term used to describe chemically-reactive molecules containing oxygen is reactive oxygen species or ROS. Two types are free radicals, such as hydroxyl, nitric oxide and superoxide, and non-radicals, such as hydrogen peroxide and lipid peroxide (Genox.com, 2010). ROS leads to oxidative damage to specific molecules which results in injury to cells or tissue. Increased production of ROS occurs as a result of a fungal or viral infection, inflammation, aging, UV radiation, pollution, excessive alcohol consumption, drug use and cigarette smoking (Genox.com, 2010).

Removal or neutralization of ROS is achieved with antioxidants – endogenous, such as catalase, glutathione and superoxide dismutase, or exogenous, such as vitamins A, C, E, bioflavonoids and carotenoids. Oxidative damage to the eye, particularly the retina and the lens, is a contributing factor to age-related macular degeneration and cataracts.

Oxidative stress is a strong determinant in how the body is functioning on a cellular level. The key to living a long and healthy life lies in understanding the mechanisms that bring about the process of cellular degradation and premature aging.

Notes

Gottschling, Barbara C. et al. "The Role of Oxidative Stress in Indium Phosphide-Induced Lung Carcinogenesis in Rats," *Toxicological Sciences*, Vol. 64, No. 1, 2001.

"What Is Oxidative Stress," Genox.com, Accessed August 1, 2010. www.genox.com/what_is_oxidative_stress.html

Chapter 24: Diabetes

Diabetes is one of the fastest growing disease processes in our times. It is the sixth leading killer in America, according to the December 2009 issue of the journal *Diabetes Care* (Huang, December 2009). By 2034, diabetes is expected to double, and the cost to treat it will triple to more than $300 billion annually.

Diabetes is divided into two types. Type 1 diabetes was previously called insulin-dependent diabetes mellitus or juvenile-onset diabetes (CDC, November 30, 2009). In type 1 diabetes, the pancreas is not able to produce proper amounts of insulin. About 10 percent of diabetics have type 1 diabetes.

Type 2 diabetes was previously called non-insulin-dependent diabetes mellitus or adult-onset diabetes (CDC, November 30, 2009). Type 2 is related to lifestyle, which includes diet, weight and exercise. With type 2 diabetes, the cells are unable to receive the insulin readily available in the bloodstream. Insulin helps to escort glucose into the cell. Every cell needs glucose to function properly. Humans must be able to properly use insulin so they can maintain normal blood sugar levels. Healthy blood sugar levels are a key to living a long fruitful life.

Managing diabetes is a billion-dollar industry when you consider the alarming number of people currently falling into this category. Doctor visits, insulin medication, testing and injection equipment, as well as surgeries, are all needed. The management of diabetes, along with many other diseases, is another example of why our nation's health care costs are so high.

The cell and insulin receptors

The American public is not being told about the true causes of diabetes that could change how this disease is understood. People have been sold on the idea that diabetes is a blood sugar regulation and insulin malfunction disorder. The insulin receptors, which lie on the cell's surface, are unable to process the glucose that is present in the bloodstream in people who have type 2 diabetes. This belief that diabetes is a blood sugar/insulin disease is similar to the idea most Americans have that cholesterol causes heart disease, despite the fact that half of the people who have a heart attack or stroke have normal cholesterol levels and some of the healthiest people have high cholesterol levels in conjunction with low systemic inflammation.

The truth about type 2 diabetes is that it is a cell wall receptor malfunction, not a blood sugar/insulin disorder. This means that the insulin receptors are malfunctioning. Insulin and glucose are available, but not able to get into the cell because the door is shut. The bi-lipid membrane that surrounds the cell, which allows insulin to enter, is not open for business. The closed sign is out as glucose looks in the window waiting for the doors to open so it can be escorted in by insulin.

A close look at the structure of the cell wall offers an explanation of why it might not be receptive to insulin, which is the key to insulin resistance. Each cell of the body has a bi-lipid layer that surrounds the cell. It is a semi-permeable membrane much like a selective filter. It allows nutrients in and waste products out. It also has receptors for various things, including insulin. The structure and function of the cell wall is the key to not only insulin and glucose uptake, but nutrient and oxygen assimilation as well. This determines how well our body functions at a cellular level. A defective cell wall is a prerequisite to illness and ultimately a short life span. This is the number one factor that causes type 2 diabetes. A healthy cell wall allows insulin, glucose and other nutrients to pass this selective barrier and deliver its goods.

The role of diet

Three important areas of concern precede type 2 diabetes. The first relates to what we eat. Most people with type 2 diabetes eat a less than desirable diet. Usually, it is high in refined oils. These are oxidized fats, the kind your body does not want. This means fried foods cooked in rancid oils such as canola, safflower, sunflower and other oils. It also includes a highly processed carbohydrate diet such as baked goods, white bread, white rice, pizza, pastries, pasta and other foods lacking in fiber. Refined sugar intake such as soda pop, candy and energy drinks can also contribute. These foods cause insulin spikes, which increases inflammation. Over time, this can cause a strain and eventually weakening of the pancreas, as well as be a major contributor to cell wall deterioration.

Cell wall construction

The second area of concern is how the cell wall is constructed, as it is a bi-lipid layer. Whatever type of fat that is consumed will end up being the construction materials for each cell wall. The body will use whatever material it is given in order to construct this precious membrane. If a house is built with inferior building materials, it will be susceptible to breakdown. Most fast foods are cooked in rancid oils that are used over and over again. Polyunsaturated oils are oxidized fats. They create free radicals (Johansen, 2005). Building a cell wall from these rancid oils will repel not only insulin, but other vital nutrients as well including glucose and oxygen. These oils cause the cell wall to lose its fluidity and become more rigid. The body becomes starved at a cellular level. It is well know that these types of oils contribute to heart disease, cancer and many other disease processes including diabetes. They also increase inflammation and trigger the body to store arterial plaque.

Inflammation

The third area of importance is inflammation. Chronic inflammation changes cell wall integrity over time. Sustained systemic heat—inflammation—hardens the cell wall, making it less permeable to nutrients including insulin. This process, like cardiovascular disease, takes years to develop into a diseased state. This book explains over and over again how chronic low-grade infection (lingering pathogens) translates into chronic systemic inflammation. Chronic inflammation leads to chronic illness.

Inflammation and diet are directly related to cell wall construction. What we need to understand is that the focus of any illness, especially diabetes, should be on the health of the cell wall. This is in sharp contrast to playing the glucose management game. Blood sugar/insulin regulation problems are the effect of an unhealthy cell wall. Treating the effect is completely ignoring the cause. A healthy cell wall allows all nutrients including insulin to cross this semi-permeable membrane and feed the cell properly. Healthy cell walls need to be built not just to prevent diabetes, but also to allow the body to function at an optimal level. The building blocks for a healthy cell wall have to do with the proper intake of healthy oils. This means omega 3 oils, which include flax and fish oils. Coconut and olive oils are also beneficial. When the diet includes these oils on a regular basis, the cell wall will use these nutrients to build a proper foundation.

Antioxidants

Research shows that the intake of antioxidants and healthy oils has a strong correlation with the reduction or elimination of diabetes (Montonen, 2004). Study after study indicates this relationship. Antioxidants reduce free radical damage and inflammation. These are two key factors that affect cell wall function.

Type 2 diabetes can be overcome if people understand that diabetes is just an effect. The main cause is chronic inflammation and a poor diet causing cell wall malformation, leading to nutrient depletion. The effect is diabetes and poor health. Most diabetic patients have other symptoms and illnesses that are also related to cell wall malfunction. Improve the cell wall, reduce inflammation and many disorders will either be greatly reduced or may go away entirely on their own. Treating the cause instead of the effect makes good sense.

Notes

"Frequently Asked Questions: Basics About Diabetes," National Center for Chronic Disease Prevention and Health, Centers for Disease Control and Prevention, Accessed November 30, 2009. www.cdc.gov/diabetes/faq/basics.htm#3

Huang, Elbert. "Projecting the Future Diabetes Population Size and Related Costs for the U.S.," *Diabetes Care*, December 2009.

Johansen, Jeanette Schultz et al. "Oxidative Stress and the Use of Antioxidants in Diabetes: Linking Basic Science to Clinical Practice," *Cardiovascular Diabetology*, Vol. 4, 2005.

Montonen, Jukka et al. "Dietary Antioxidant Intake and Risk of Type 2 Diabetes," *Diabetes Care*, Vol. 27, No. 2, 2004.

References

Kaneto, Hideaki. "Beneficial Effects of Antioxidants in Diabetes: Possible Protection of Pancreatic b-Cells Against Glucose Toxicity," *Diabetes*, Vol. 48, December 1999.

Kaufmann, Doug A. with David Holland, M.D. *Infectious Diabetes*. Rockwall, Texas: MediaTrition Inc., 2003.

Parker, Lester, Ed., et al. *Antioxidant Diabetes Management*. New York: Marcel Dekker Inc., 2000.

"Well-Defined Quantity of Antioxidants in Diet Can Improve Insulin Resistance, Study Finds," ScienceDaily, June 22, 2010. www.sciencedaily.com/releases/2010/06/100621091205.htm

Chapter 25: Cardiovascular Disease

Some information on cardiovascular disease is covered in Chapter 14 on Chronic Inflammation. However, I wanted to touch on some key points that were not mentioned in that chapter.

The role of pathogens

Lingering pathogens create strokes, heart disease, damaging cholesterol, heart attacks and poor low-density lipoprotein (LDL) to high-density lipoproteins (HDL) ratios. In 2000, a major study led by Paul Ridker, M.D., on inflammation markers in predicting cardiovascular disease was conducted at Harvard University. This study came to the conclusion that systemic inflammation is a major indicator in contributing to high cholesterol, poor HDL to LDL ratios and cardiovascular disease. Of the major markers measured, researchers found that a high level of C-reactive protein was the strongest predictor of the risk of cardiovascular events (Ridker, December 2000). The study was well publicized nationally and reported on major news networks. However, to this day, this study has made little headway on the extensive use of statin drugs, which continue to be the recommended protocol by most physicians.

Basic mechanism of cardiovascular disease

A few years ago, several research papers were published from studies, and now several books and magazine articles have been published, pointing to lingering pathogens and chronic infection as being the underlying cause of cardiovascular disease.

Pathogenic entry into the heart and coronary arteries comes from three specific areas that are proximally related to the heart. First are the lungs that sit on both sides of the heart and exchange blood directly. Next is the mouth, which is a natural harbor for bacterial infection. This infection can leak down into the blood and lymph fluid directly into the heart area. Third is the stomach, which sits directly below the heart. Bacteria can back up from the stomach into the esophagus and then invade the heart area.

These three areas can harbor lingering pathogens that can be transported into the heart and coronary arteries leading to chronic infection. The stage can then be set for this whole cardiovascular inflammatory process to unfold. Once a bacterium, for instance, sets up residence in your artery, a call goes out for your immune system to respond to this invasion, as your white blood cells recognize this presence. The white blood cells go into action by attacking the pathogenic invader wherever it is. The way the immune system attacks causes small holes in the endothelial lining (tissue that lines body organs and cavities) of the artery. It is like shooting bullets into the inner lining of the arterial wall, which leave their marks. This persistent attack will cause damage and subsequent inflammation to occur on the inner artery wall. This initial damage sets up the scenario that brings about long-term, low-grade inflammation. The inflammation becomes the effect that carries out much of the future damage.

Bacteria

Specific bacteria have been proven to be some of the main culprits in causing this chronic condition. The primary bacterial invaders are *Chlamydia pneumoniae*, *Helicobacter pylori*, *Streptococcus mutans*, *Streptococcus pneumoniae* and *Staphylococcus aureus*. *Chlamydia pneumoniae* is the most publicized and pathologically documented bacterium involved in heart disease. *Chlamydia pneumoniae* is the number one cause of cardiovascular disease, according to *The Heart Attack Germ*, a book by Louis Dvonch, M.D., and Russell Dvonch, as well as other supporting literature. The reason for this has to do with many factors that are well documented in this informative book. For starters, *Chlamydia pneumoniae* has the tendency to invade endothelial tissue. *Chlamydia pneumoniae* prefers to adhere to the mucosal lining of the lungs causing pneumonia, as well as the inner lining of the blood vessels causing vascular disease. It adheres not only to this type of tissue, but it also seems to prefer arterial plaque, as it has the ability to soak up cholesterol. The other factor involves its ability to enter monocytes and lymphocytes, two types of white blood cells. *Chlamydia pneumoniae* can create a membrane around itself for protection, once inside these host cells. This bug can either become latent for a period of time or start the replication process (Dvonch, 2003).

When pathogens start invading the arterial lining of blood vessels, they start to fire up the inflammatory process. Damaged arterial cells secrete a substance called arachidonic acid. White blood cells are attracted to this substance. Cytokines and leukotrienes, chemical mediators, also start attracting white blood cells to the area. The increase in immune attacks greatly increases free radical activity and damage. Free radicals oxidize the cholesterol, changing it from the HDL form to the oxidized LDL form, much like olive oil does if left exposed to light and heat. This oxidated effect then damages cell wall structures. Monocytes are white blood cells that turn to macrophages as they enter the artery. They are part of this army that comes swarming down to the site of injury. The first problem is that the *Chlamydia pneumoniae* have invaded the macrophages and are being escorted to the injury site with the macrophages providing the free ride. This is how the white blood cells can spread *Chlamydia pneumoniae* within the circulatory system, and throughout the entire body (BBC Online Network, February 25, 1999).

Helicobacter pylori, known more for its reputation to cause ulcers, can also rise upward from the stomach to infect the heart. Three separate studies in 1999 done by Italian, French and Polish researchers found a direct correlation between heart disease and *Helicobacter pylori* infection. *Staphylococcus aureus*, *Streptococcus mutans* and *Streptococcus pneumoniae* are other common bacteria that have been indicated in heart disease. The heart itself is composed mostly of muscle tissue that is fairly resistant to damage. However, the heart valves are delicate feather-like structures that allow blood to enter the heart. Lingering bacteria, such as the common ones mentioned above, can infect these delicate valves and with the help of chronic inflammation can cause irreversible damage. This is why there are so many heart valve replacements today. The valve becomes fibrotic in nature and loses its ability to open and close properly, thereby causing a leaky valve.

Staphylococcus aureus is the most common resistive and invasive bacteria of our time. Though it prefers the sinus cavities, it can easily invade the heart and its vascular structures. *Streptococcus pneumoniae* loves the lungs and, much like its counterpart, can easily invade cardiovascular structures from its closely related anatomical perch. Most dentists understand general mouth bacteria, especially *Streptococcus mutans*, as a primary cause of gum and heart disease. Most physicians and cardiologists do recognize gum infection, especially with *Staph* and *Strep*, as being primary risks in heart disease.

Viruses

Several well known viruses can also be involved such as cytomegalovirus (CMV), herpes simplex virus (HSV) and respiratory syncytialvirus (RSV). CMV has received most of the attention for its ability to be a factor in patients who have cardiovascular disease (Dvonch, 2003).

A study in 2000 by the Heart, Lung and Blood Institute found subjects that had the highest levels of immune system antibodies to CMV had a 76 percent greater chance of developing heart disease over five years, compared to the ones who had the lowest levels or none at all. Other studies have also shown a significant connection as well. HSV has also been linked to cardiovascular disease. A study in 2000 from Finland showed that patients infected with HSV were twice as likely to die from heart attack and had double the risk for cardiovascular disease.

I mentioned in Chapter 32 on Respiratory Disorders that RSV is a primary causative factor in chronic bronchitis. Though no significant studies were administered connecting this virus to cardiovascular disease, there may be a secondary inflammatory effect that plays a role in this germ's ability to proliferate the inflammatory process. Because the lungs are so closely connected both anatomically and through direct circulatory connections to the heart, inflammation in the lungs and bronchial tubes will have a secondary inflammatory reaction within the heart and its circulatory structures. Respiratory tract infection/inflammation not only contribute to heart inflammation, but also to systemic inflammation as well, as the blood is being continually heated up as it passes through the lung area. RSV seems to be much more prevalent today than in years past. This virus creates a tremendous amount of heat when active. The typical chronic dry cough with this virus is an effect of this heat.

Other research has pointed to mycoplasma and *Candida albicans* infections as possible factors in cardiovascular disease. Because mycoplasmas have some of the same characteristics that *Chlamydia pneumoniae* exhibits in its ability to replicate inside a cell, take over lymphocytes and stimulate the inflammatory process, this makes a strong case for this bug's involvement in heart disease. *Candida albicans* is slow moving as most fungi are. Some cases of heart valve disease may be rooted with *Candida albicans* infestation, though plaque formation may also be an effect.

HDL to LDL ratios

How the molecular structure of HDL to LDL ratios change is related to the amount of sustained heat that is generated within the circulatory system over time. As I have previously mentioned, this is like taking a fresh bottle of olive oil and exposing it to the sun and heat over a period of time. The oil changes its molecular structure by oxidizing and becoming rancid. Oxidizing means that it has increased its free radicals. This is the same effect that happens when you have systemic inflammation. Sustained low-grade heat over time lends itself to cholesterol in the arteries turning to an oxidized form. This form then creates the increase of LDLs and lowering of HDLs. The bloodstream is a large enclosed tube that will respond to distant stimuli within the enclosure. This means that any lingering pathogens that contribute to systemic inflammation, even though they may lie far from the heart area, should be considered as secondary pathogenic contributors to overall cardiovascular disease, due to their warming effect within this tube-like structure.

Testing for C-reactive protein levels is an indicator of inflammation and infection. High levels are indicated in chronic inflammatory conditions as well as possible cardiovascular disease. High homocysteine levels are also an indicator of higher risks for heart attacks and strokes. Homocysteine levels rise in conjunction with high inflammatory levels, as well as with high protein diets. This amino acid combines with LDL cholesterol to form a substance that greatly irritates arterial walls. It also can contribute to higher LDL levels. Increased immune attacks cause increases in free radicals within the artery. Free radicals are known for their ability to damage tissue. High levels of LDL cholesterol, damaged arterial lining, elevated homocysteine, attacking immune cells, chemical mediators, free radicals, pathogens and the inflammatory effects they cause continue to damage the endothelial tissue. Arterial plaque is then formed in this response to heal the damaged lining. This plaque forms a patch over the scar. This scab is a structurally weak patch that can break off at any time due to circulatory stress and cause a stroke or heart attack. Inflammation keeps perpetuating more inflammation as the damage continues on.

A slow process

The problem is that this process is a slow forming and mostly a hidden asymptomatic pattern that takes years to reach a symptomatic level. Lingering pathogens, poor diet and high stress, with little or no exercise, set in motion this disease process.

Notes

"Chlamydia Linked to Heart Disease," BBC Online Network, February 25, 1999. news.bbc.co.uk/hi/english/health/newsid_285000/285757.stm

Dvonch, Louis, M.D., and Russell Dvonch. *The Heart Attack Germ: Prevent Strokes, Heart Attacks, and the Symptoms of Alzheimer's by Protecting Yourself From the Infections and Inflammation of Cardiovascular Disease*. New York: Writer's Showcase, 2003.

Ridker, Paul, M.D., et al. "C-Reactive Protein and Other Markers of Inflammation in the Prediction of Cardiovascular Disease in Women," *New England Journal of Medicine*, December 2000.

References

Bowman, Lee. "Blood Test Can Predict a Cardiovascular Event," *Seattle Post-Intelligencer*, January 10, 2007.

"C-Reactive Protein Test to Screen for Heart Disease: Why Do We Need Another?" Harvard Health Publications, Harvard Medical School, Accessed June 7, 2007.

www.health.harvard.edu/newsweek/C-Reactive_Protein_test_to_screen_for_heart_disease.htm

Candidiasis: Pathogenesis, Diagnosis, and Treatment. New York: Raven Press Ltd., 1993.

Cromie, William J. "Better Way to Predict Heart Attacks Is Discovered," Harvard University Gazette, March 23, 2000.
www.hno.harvard.edu/gazette/2000/03.23/heart.html

Cromie, William J. "Inflammation May Forecast Heart Attacks," Harvard University Gazette, February 12, 1998.
www.hno.harvard.edu/gazette/1998/02.12/InflammationMay.html

Dorsainvil, Pierre A., M.D. "Cardiobacterium," eMedicine, Accessed June 26, 2005.
www.emedicine.com/med/topic284.htm

Gronczewski, Craig A., M.D. "Clostridium Difficile Colitis," eMedicine, Accessed March 9, 2005.
www.emedicine.com/MED/topics3412.htm

Hallum, J.L. and T.W. Williams, Jr. "Candida Endocarditis." In G.P. Bodey (ed.), *Candidiasis: Pathogenesis, Diagnosis, and Treatment.* New York: Raven Press Ltd., 1993.

Liebman, Bonnie. "CRP: Another Piece of the Heart-Disease Puzzle?" *Nutrition Action Healthletter*, March 2003.

Nicolson, Garth L., Ph.D. "Chronic Infectious Diseases," The Institute for Molecular Medicine," Accessed June 26, 2005.
www.immed.org/illness/fatigue_illness_research.html

Ojcius, David M., Toni Darville and Patrick M. Bavoil. "Can Chlamydia Be Stopped?" *Scientific American*, May 2005.

Pelletier, Lawrence, Jr., M.D. "Infective Endocarditis," eMedicine, Accessed June 8, 2005.
www.emedicine.com/MED/topic671.htm

Chapter 26: Cholesterol

Cholesterol, a waxy substance made up of sterols and fatty acids, is important to how the brain and body function. Every cell in the body contains cholesterol. It has many purposes, such as being a precursor to hormone production. This includes the sex hormones testosterone, estrogen and progesterone. Cholesterol also helps produce corticosteroids, which help to reduce inflammation and promote healing. Cholesterol is needed for proper nerve functioning, especially in the brain. Vitamin D and even bile need cholesterol for production. Every cell membrane has a lipid bilayer that requires fat for proper functioning.

Cholesterol drugs

Tampering with the body's cholesterol production will affect other systems of the body as well, creating potential cascading metabolic imbalances. Statin drugs reduce cholesterol production in the liver. The body actually becomes cholesterol deficient. When people understand how statins work and tax various body systems, they can then make an informed decision about taking them based on scientific research.

A *Business Week* cover story called "Do Cholesterol Drugs Do Any Good?" examined research on the effectiveness of statins such as Lipitor (Carey, January 28, 2008). Therapeutics Initiative, a government-funded organization whose purpose is to study data on drugs and determine how well they work, analyzed evidence from years of trials with statins. They found no benefit in people over the age of 65, no matter how much their cholesterol declined, and no benefit in women of any age. No overall reduction in total deaths or illnesses requiring hospitalization occurred despite big reductions in bad cholesterol.

"Most people are taking something with no chance of benefit and a risk of harm," James Wright, M.D., director of Therapeutics Initiative and a professor at the University of British Columbia, was quoted as saying in the article. On side effects, ten to 15 percent of all statin users suffer from them including cognitive impairment, sexual dysfunction and muscle pain, Dr. Wright added (Carey, January 28, 2008).

Beatrice Golomb, M.D., associate professor at the University of California at San Diego School of Medicine, also stated that the widespread use of statins comes at the cost of billions of dollars a year, not just for the drugs, but cholesterol screening, visits and other tests. Rodney A. Hayward, M.D., professor of internal medicine at the University of Michigan Medical School, said, "It is almost impossible to find someone who believes in statins who does not get a lot of money from the industry" (Carey, January 28, 2008).

Drug manufacturers make sure the researchers and doctors who extol the benefits of medications are well compensated. The article discusses how in other cultures cholesterol levels are not directly related to heart disease, just as it is becoming apparent in ours as well. It explains how people can become fixated on markers for health assessment without understanding the significance of the marker in relationship to their health. Cholesterol testing and treatment have not been the solution to heart disease because they were based on false premises (Carey, January 28, 2008).

Heart disease and inflammation

The Cholesterol Conspiracy by Ladd R. McNamara, M.D., 2003, analyzes studies on cholesterol and heart disease and exposes conflicts of interest within the industry in promoting statins. The original book, with the same title, was written by Edward R. Pinckney, M.D., former co-editor of the Journal of the American Medical Association, and Russell L. Smith, M.D., in 1991.

Here are key points from the book, which present concepts on cholesterol and heart disease:

- Atherosclerosis is a disease characterized primarily by inflammation of the arterial lining caused by oxidative damage from homocysteine.
- Homocysteine combined with other free radicals and toxins oxidizes arteries and LDL cholesterol, which in turn releases C-reactive protein, a marker for an inflammatory response of the arteries.
- This is the beginning of plaque buildup and ultimately cardiovascular disease.

"LDL cholesterol only becomes bad when it is damaged by oxidative free radicals," Dr. McNamara said in his book. "Only the damaged or oxidized form of LDL cholesterol sticks to the arterial walls to initiate the formation of plaque. LDL cholesterol is not bad, it is critical to maintain life. Therefore, it is critical to realize that it is not simply the level of LDL cholesterol that is the issue; it is actually the level of oxidized or damaged cholesterol that is of greater concern. The combination of damaged LDL cholesterol and a damaged arterial lining is what causes LDL cholesterol to stick to the arteries, whether or not the LDL cholesterol level is normal or not" (McNamara, 2003).

Arterial plaque contains very little, if any, saturated fat. Omega-6 and cholesterol are the most abundant components of clogged arteries. When they are in an oxidized form, which is the effect of inflammation and free radical damage, then they become lethal in an artery (Peskin, June 2008).

I have stated in this book that inflammation is the key to cardiovascular disease. Dr. McNamara's book confirms everything that I believe and have written about this subject. His understanding of this disease process is very accurate.

However, the main source of the inflammation is the key to truly understanding this whole picture. Lingering pathogens are responsible for creating much of the inflammation, which in turn creates the oxidative damage to the LDL cholesterol. Free radical damage from other unhealthy lifestyle patterns such as smoking, drugs, excessive alcohol intake, poor nutrition, stress and other factors can definitely contribute to the overall picture. Remember, pathogens cause free radicals to form as a byproduct of immune attacks on the lingering pathogens, and this keeps stimulating the ongoing inflammatory process. The process then creates increased homocysteine and raises C-reactive protein markers. Dr. McNamara stresses the importance of B_6, B_{12}, folic acid and various antioxidants to keep homocysteine levels down. This is valuable information, but does not address the pathogenic factor. I believe those fortunate people who have few or no lingering pathogens in their systems, especially in their coronary arteries, will have a healthy cardiovascular system because they have less inflammation. Antioxidants and B vitamins are helpful to those with lingering pathogens or an unhealthy lifestyle as they help counter the increased homocysteine levels and inflammation.

Statin drugs

Statins do possess some ability to lower inflammation. However, that may be their only value. This small benefit comes at a steep price financially and at the expense of patients' overall long-term health. Taking statins results in a long list of serious symptoms, according to research. They include:

- Mental and visual impairment.
- Neurological damage.
- Memory loss.
- Hormone reduction causing sexual and brain dysfunction.
- Mood disturbances.
- Mild to severe depression.
- Fatigue.

- Immune dysfunction.
- Heart failure.
- Cancer risk increase.
- Skeletal muscle and connective tissue dysfunction and damage.
- Muscle twitching, spasms and muscle weakness.
- Liver dysfunction and possible liver damage.
- Constipation.

Statins also deplete the body's supply of coenzyme Q10. This vital antioxidant is a major component of the Krebs Cycle, which is the body's main energy production system. This often is why fatigue immediately sets in when patients start taking statin drugs. A lack of coenzyme Q10 can also weaken the heart, which requires high amounts of this enzyme to function properly.

The longer a patient is on statin drugs the greater chance that a long-term illness may occur. Many patients' symptoms are not being attributed to the statins because of failure of the patient to know and identify the side effects, and failure of the doctor to associate the symptoms with statin drugs. In addition, many of these patients are also on other medications, which may have overlapping symptoms. The symptoms caused by the statins are often treated with other drugs, which may cause other symptoms as well. At some point, it becomes almost impossible to know what drug is causing which symptom. From my research, I believe that almost everyone on statin drugs experiences some of the above side effects. Doctors are routinely ignoring and/or not reporting the side effects. I think the reports that side effects occur in only 10 to 15 percent of people who take statins are very misleading.

A patient of mine has been on statin drugs for eight years. He came in complaining of problems with the coordination and movement of three of his fingers. He could not straighten out his fingers much of the time and had problems closing them as well. His partner also reported that he felt very tired much of the time and could hardly get out of a chair due to pain and stiffness. These symptoms occurred since he had been on the drugs. Several sessions of acupuncture resulted in little improvement. When he told me he had been on a popular statin drug for eight years, I suggested that maybe the statin drug was responsible for the finger problems. Finger movement has both neurological and skeletal components. These two systems are greatly affected by statin drugs. It seemed logical that this could be the culprit. I told him to go back to the doctor that was prescribing the drugs and mention to him about the side effects he was having. When he returned, he said he questioned the doctor about the finger problems and the need to take the cholesterol drugs in the first place as he had read the *Business Week* article.

The doctor's response was interesting. First, the doctor did not think there was a correlation between my patient's muscular skeletal problems and the statin drug he had been on for eight years. Then his doctor said, "We can't do much for diabetes, but we got it right with our cholesterol drugs." He then wrote my friend a different prescription for another statin drug, which was the same drug that was mentioned in the *Business Week* article. The study on this drug showed a decrease in cholesterol. However, the coronary arteries actually increased in plaque formation on this combination drug during the trial study.

The side effects of statin drugs

The symptoms at the top of the list as possible side effects from statin drugs are muscle weakness, stiffness, pain, mental impairment and fatigue. A rational conclusion could be made that there may be a connection between the drug and the symptoms my patient experienced. A commonsense approach would have been to take him off the drugs for at least a month to see if the finger problems and fatigue would improve.

The eye-opening statement the doctor made was, "We got it right with our cholesterol drugs." Where did his research come from to make such a statement? Doctors are brainwashed by the system to promote what sells. They have little awareness that no viable studies exist proving that these toxic drugs actually reduce death rates from heart disease and strokes. The education for doctors is mainly coming from drug company sales representatives that constantly parade in and out of their offices. Do you think the sales people are going to show doctors this data? Many of the statin studies were funded by pharmaceutical companies hoping desperately to get favorable outcomes to back why millions of Americans should be taking the drugs. There should have been clearly defined data showing some kind of positive relationship between reduced cholesterol levels and death from heart attacks and strokes. The purpose for taking these drugs in the first place was to save lives. What is the value of lowering cholesterol if it does not do at least that one thing?

Another person I know who has been on statin drugs for eight years has lost much of her cognitive function and has severe fatigue. She presented the information from the *Business Week* article to her doctor. His response was that this information had not made its way to the doctors as yet. Until it does, she should keep taking the statins. He also ignored the relationship between her symptoms and the drugs.

The important Harvard studies

Maybe the Harvard Medical School study on the role of inflammation in heart disease, which was widely reported in the media and medical journals in 2000, also has not made its way down to the doctors (Ridker, March 23, 2000).

In both cases I have described, the prescribing physicians ignored the obvious statin-related symptoms in favor of staying the statin course. I have spoken with many other patients who had severe reactions and felt terrible soon after beginning to take statin drugs. Their doctors were all very upset with them for dropping the medication. I seriously doubt that even 10 percent of all statin-related symptoms are being reported by doctors. What is more likely true is that over 90 percent of all users are probably experiencing one or more acute side effects. Then there are long-term health effects that will appear years later.

Harvard's initial study discovered that inflammation, as measured by the marker C-reactive protein, is a very potent predictor for cardiovascular disease (Ridker, April 3, 1997). Another Harvard study showed that C-reactive protein appeared to be a much stronger predictor of future heart attack risk than LDL cholesterol (Ridker, March 23, 2000). However, seeing inflammation as a cause is shortsighted because it fails to consider why inflammation exists in the first place. Inflammation's root cause again is lingering pathogens and subsequent free radical damage. This translates in traditional medical terms as a chronic infection. Eliminating pathogens and their subsequent infection results in the substantial reduction of inflammation. Free radicals also need to be reduced in conjunction with pathogen removal. Free radicals are created in response to chronic infections and inflammation as well as other lifestyle factors.

Cardiologist Paul Ridker, associate professor of medicine at Harvard University, has been the lead researcher for much of the well-documented and publicized research on inflammation and heart disease. Dr. Ridker has stated that nearly half of all heart attacks occur among men and women with normal cholesterol levels. The amount of risk associated with high sensitivity C-reactive protein is almost twice that associated with high levels of low density lipoprotein (Crombie, 2000). What Dr. Ridker is saying is that LDL cholesterol levels are not that valuable in terms of determining the risk of heart attacks and strokes.

Statins have been shown to reduce the enzyme rho-kinase. This seems to help lower inflammation in the arteries. When looking at why a person has heart disease, the focus should shift to reducing inflammation, which is what causes heart disease. This would explain the slight improvement in those who had this preexisting condition when using statins. Inflammation, which caused the heart disease, was already present and statins did help to reduce the inflammation that in turn helped reduce the progression of heart disease. This slight reduction in inflammation, though, comes at a high price as potential side effects and exuberant costs seem to greatly outweigh these gains. The University of Michigan's Rodney A. Hayward, M.D., said in the *Business Week* article that "current evidence supports ignoring LDL cholesterol altogether." Jerome R. Hoffman, M.D., professor of clinical Medicine at the University of California at Los Angeles, stated, "The way our health care runs, it is not based on data, it is based on what makes money" (Carey, January 28, 2008).

Drug companies and illness

"Suddenly Sick: The Hidden Big Business Behind Your Doctors Diagnosis," an article published in *The Seattle Times* on June 26, 2005, was a special report on how the drug industry influences what constitutes disease, who has it and how it should be treated. By changing key markers for cholesterol, hypertension, diabetes and weight with little scientific evidence to support the changes, the drug companies were then able to create new patients by placing 75 percent of the U.S. population under one of the above changed guidelines (Kelleher, June 26, 2005).

Cholesterol markers came down from 240 or above to 220 or above. This seemingly small change added 42.6 million people to the new definition. Blood pressure guidelines were also lowered from above 160/100 to 140/90. This added an extra 13.5 million more people to the mix (Kelleher, June 26, 2005).

This lengthy report gives details about how big business is so powerful that it can make major changes in medical guidelines despite clear evidence to the contrary, or at least, little evidence to support these changes. The new cholesterol and blood pressure guidelines were promoted by physicians to the unsuspecting public as parameters for their revised treatment approach. Television and newspaper ads helped to fortify this mindset to millions of people who were convinced that there was some scientific basis for these changes.

Why are doctors still to this day still singing the "Let's All Lower Our Cholesterol by Taking Statins" fight song, despite the clear evidence that reducing cholesterol by taking these drugs is not very beneficial in terms of preventing heart disease and strokes? Could they be possibly ignoring the scientific research in favor of marketing the statins?

The much publicized Harvard studies, the in-depth investigation by *The Seattle Times*, *The Cholesterol Conspiracy* book and the *Business Week* cover story give strong evidence about the problems with statins and cholesterol. There seems to be not only a huge discrepancy about the role cholesterol actually plays in causing heart attacks and strokes, but of even more concern is the use of expensive and toxic drugs to lower cholesterol, which may not be nearly as threatening as the drug companies led Americans to believe. A major political agenda seemed to play a role in this whole scheme. Huge financial gains were to be made by certain interest groups that were well invested in promoting the idea that cholesterol is the culprit and something must be done about it; lower cholesterol by buying our dangerous and expensive drugs.

About four years ago I had an acquaintance, a retired drug salesman, who mentioned to me that he would love to come out of retirement so he could get in on the huge profits that the drug companies were making from these new drugs. He mentioned that he had several doctor friends who had left their practices to become drug salesman in order to get in on the feeding frenzy. He said these drugs are very cheap to manufacture, and the markup is phenomenal.

The special report in *The Seattle Times* states that pharmaceutical companies have commandeered the process by which diseases are defined (Kelleher, June 26, 2005). Many decision makers at the World Health Organization, the U.S. National Institutes of Health and some of America's most prestigious medical societies take money from the drug companies and then promote the industry's agenda, according to *The Times* article. Some diseases have been radically redefined without much basis in medical evidence. The tactic of targeting younger and healthier people by narrowing the parameters of what constitutes sickness creates a whole new population of patients. The end result of these business practices is skyrocketing sales of prescription drugs, increasing numbers of medical testing and visits, and soaring health care costs. Worst of all, millions of people who are taking these drugs may end up with other symptoms, as well as possible long-term health risks. These symptoms are often treated with other drugs. The treatment may not only make people sick, but could eventually kill them (Kelleher, June 26, 2005).

The role of antioxidants and phytonutrients

It is not much of a stretch to understand that statins are not the answer for cardiovascular disease. Anti-inflammatories are a better choice, however, they are not the best choice as they, too, have side effects. At least they are reducing inflammation, which treats more of the root cause of heart disease. The best choice is to increase your intake of antioxidants. Comprehensive research shows that they reduce free radical damage and have strong antioxidant and anti-inflammatory effects. In addition, they support immune function, slow the aging process and may prevent other serious illnesses, including cancer. Many studies have confirmed these benefits. See Chapter 11: Antioxidants and Phytonutrients to get the full picture.

Research important

After reading this chapter, it would be easy to come to the conclusion that big money is driving the cholesterol push, not science. Americans are still being swayed in this direction as the medical system, which is promoting statins to the tune of billions of dollars in revenue each year, has not yet read the current research. People have been conditioned to associate cholesterol with heart disease. This has been beat into the public by all the so-called experts people look up to, as well as the media, which are well compensated in promoting traditional medicine's agenda. The unaware American public trusts that the medical system has done its research. This is what happens when big business makes health decisions for people. Doing research allows people to come from a place of educated awareness. This way they can stay in charge of their own health. Self knowledge allows people to see a clearer picture, which enables them to make effective decisions based on research and sound judgment instead of hype and intimidation.

Notes

Carey, John. "Do Cholesterol Drugs Do Any Good?" *Business Week*, January 28, 2008.

"C-Reactive Protein Test to Screen for Heart Disease: Why Do We Need Another Test?" Harvard Health Publications, Harvard Medical School, Accessed June 7, 2007.
www.health.harvard.edu/newsweek/C-Reactive_Protein_test_to_screen_for_heart_disease.htm

Crombie, William J. "Better Way to Predict Heart Attacks Is Discovered," Harvard University Gazette, March 23, 2000.
www.hno.harvard.edu/gazette/2000/03.23/heart.html

Kelleher, Susan and Duff Wilson. "Suddenly Sick: The Hidden Big Business Behind Your Doctors Diagnosis," *The Seattle Times*, June 26, 2005.

McNamara, Ladd R., M.D. *The Cholesterol Conspiracy*, OrthoMolecular Medicine Inc., 2003.

Peskin, Brian Scott. "Vytorin Failure Explained–A New View of LDL," *Townsend Letter*, June 2008.

Ridker, Paul M., M.D. et al. "C-reactive Protein and Other Markers of Inflammation in the Prediction of Cardiovascular Disease in Women," *New England Journal of Medicine*, Vol. 342, March 23, 2000.

Ridker, Paul M., M.D. et al. "Inflammation, Aspirin, and the Risk of Cardiovascular Disease in Apparently Healthy Men," *New England Journal of Medicine*, Vol. 336, April 3, 1997.

References

Faloon, William. "Consumers Misled About Cholesterol and Statin Drugs," *Life Extension*, May 2008.

Kaslow, Jemery. *Cardiovascular Efficiency vs. Nutritional Deficiency*, Accessed June 21, 2008.
www.drkaslow.com/html/cholesterol.htm

Libby, Peter. "Inflammation and Cardiovascular Disease Mechanisms," *American Journal of Clinical Nutrition*, Vol. 83, No. 2, February 2006.

"New Studies Confirm Lethal Effects of Elevated C-Reactive Protein," *Life Extension*, May 2008.

Stein, Rob. "Inflammation May Impair Heart as Much as Cholesterol," *Washington Post*, January 6, 2005.

Weatherby, Craig. "Inflammation, Cardiovascular Disease, and Omega-3s: Research Confirms Damaging Interaction Between Cholesterol and Inflammation," Vital Choices, Accessed June 23, 2008.
www.imakenews.com/vitalchoiceseafood/e_article000389895.cfm?x=b4LM1Mf,blp TrCB7,w

Zhang, Weijian, M.D., Ph.D. "The Role of Lipoic Acid in Inflammation and Atherosclerosis," Linus Pauling Institute Research Report, Accessed March 13, 2008. lpi.oregonstate.edu/ss03/lipoicacid.html

Chapter 27: Intestinal Disorders

For many years people have been plagued by a number of both digestive and elimination problems. These problems are easy to explain. Constipation is usually too much heat in the intestinal tract. The heat can come from several sources. Chinese medicine would look at the diet and possibly say that heat-producing ingestants, such as too much meat and alcohol consumption, could be a factor, as both are warming. Poor spleen and kidney function will hinder the body's cooling mechanism. Liver qi stagnation, or liver fire, can also contribute to intestinal heat as the liver heat can invade the stomach, intestines and spleen. Using acupuncture and herbs to reduce the heat and balance the meridian flow, along with diet guidelines, may help immensely.

The role of pathogens

Heat is also created by various intestinal pathogens that linger in the intestinal tract. These pathogens can adhere to the mucosa lining of the intestines and feed off the nutrients that are passing by. Parasites such as *Blastocystis hominis*, *Entamoeba histolytica*, *Dientamoeba fragilis*, *Giardia*, and a host of others can invade the intestinal tract and live there for years, causing chronic inflammation and heat. They can also damage the intestinal walls leading to leaky gut syndrome. Bacteria such as *Helicobacter pylori*, *Klebsiella*, *Clostridium difficile*, *Citrobacter*, *E. coli*, *Salmonella* and *Mycobacterium paratuberculosis* can do much the same. *Helicobacter pylori* is considered the most common cause of ulcers. Viruses, mycoplasmas, mycobacteria, the spirochete that causes Lyme disease and fungi can also invade and linger as well. *Candida albicans*, *Clostridium difficile* and *E. coli* are normal inhabitants of intestinal flora in a healthy person. These can get out of control and become pathogenic following repeated antibiotic and steroid use, as well as the various drugs now commonly prescribed for gastroesophageal reflux disease. This can create severe diarrhea, as well as many other more serious symptoms and conditions. *Mycobacterium paratuberculosis* has been reported in several research studies as a prime candidate in chronic inflammatory intestinal disorders.

Medical terms such as irritable bowel syndrome, Crohn's disease, colitis, ulcerative colitis, acid reflux disease and ulcers all refer to some type of inflammation in the intestinal tract. The medical model acknowledges that *Helicobacter pylori* is a prime cause of ulcers, but somehow fails to make the connection with various other well-known organisms residing elsewhere in the intestinal tract. Basically, these diseases are just a chronic inflammatory process somewhere in the digestive tract. If bacteria can cause inflammation in the stomach, then why are the causes of these medically termed syndromes such a mystery?

Chronic inflammatory processes

A new phenomenon called gastroesophageal reflux disease (GERD) is often featured in advertisements for medication. We can hardly get through an evening of television without getting many reminders of this disease. A quick review of anatomy shows us that the only thing that divides the esophagus from the stomach is a sphincter. It cannot be such a stretch to understand that the same bacteria that causes ulcers, or another bacterium, could easily be located at the upper end of the stomach and cause inflammation in the area of this sphincter. *Helicobacter pylori*, *Shigella*, *Salmonella* and *E. coli*, as well as a host of others, can infect this sphincter and cause this labeled syndrome.

Many people are diagnosed with GERD and put on a medicine that they take daily for the rest of their lives, without ever being tested for *Helicobacter pylori*, or any of these other pathogens. To make matters worse, these medicines have several long-term side effects that are not even mentioned to patients. What these drugs do is destroy acid in the stomach and esophagus. When you destroy stomach acid, you have three problems. One is that your food particles, especially the proteins, can pass through the stomach without being properly broken down. This greatly affects the absorption of nutrients. Secondly, the purpose of stomach acid is to help kill any pathogens, such as bacteria, parasites and viruses, which are introduced into your intestinal tract. Guess what happens when this natural defense is stripped away? You have a much higher chance of allowing pathogens into the interior of the body. The third reason is because stomach acid helps keep the intestinal balance of good bugs to bad bugs in check. *Clostridium difficile* is a prime example of a normal intestinal inhabitant that is becoming infectious in some people who are put on GERD drugs.

Taking drugs that are prescribed for this newly discovered gastroesophageal reflux disease will change your entire gastrointestinal environment for the worse. You may get temporary symptom relief from these medications. However, this relief may come at the expense of setting yourself up for much more serious problems in the future. This is a prime example of how chasing symptoms around the body is such a shortsighted and potentially costly approach.

Some of the other syndromes mentioned above are considered autoimmune diseases. The truth is the immune system is going after these microbes in order to destroy them. That is its job, to destroy bugs. The immune system is doing exactly what it is supposed to be doing. The problem is that these bugs can become so deeply entrenched in the mucosa lining of the intestines that the immune system fails to root them out, but continues to try. These are termed lingering pathogens. They entered the system at some point and have found a comfortable home and do not want to leave. They are feasting on your food and nutrients. The inflammation is a direct result of the immune system's constant attacks on these microbes, as well as the heat created by just having them exist and continuing to damage healthy tissue. Toxic byproducts released during the attacks intensify the inflammation. The heat and inflammation is nothing more than an effect. The syndrome then, is a category of a symptom, which arises out of these effects. The diagnosis of irritable bowel syndrome is just an effect and nothing more. The key is not to just treat the symptom, which might be to take a laxative for constipation, a painkiller for the pain, an anti-inflammatory for the inflammation or even a steroid to reduce the immune system's attacks. These types of treatments will only reduce the effect but still leave the underlying cause. True healing comes when the invading pathogens are eliminated, so the immune system will not have a reason to attack and normal bowel function can return. If this faulty condition continues, then permanent damage can result.

Allergies and sensitivities

Allergies and sensitivities can trigger intestinal dysfunction, as well. Allergies affect meridian flow in the body. Since most meridians are associated with a particular organ, sensitivity to wheat, for instance, may cause a disruption of energy flow to the large intestine meridian, which may produce diarrhea. Another example might be a sensitivity to the mineral calcium, which is in so many foods and supplements. This could cause a disruption of energy flow to the stomach meridian. You may notice you feel nauseous when taking a calcium supplement, but do not realize that this wonderful mineral is not compatible with your stomach's meridian flow. Many people have an intolerance to gluten, which can be a major contributor. They are told that they must avoid gluten foods, which include most of the grains for the rest of their lives. Wheat and corn are common foods that can cause intestinal disturbances. A skilled practitioner can accomplish a sensitivity repatterning for any of these substances.

Most intestinal disorders have two things at the source. Intestinal pathogens and food allergies are usually the key players. The pathogens create a low-grade inflammatory process much like a low simmering fire, while the food sensitivities represent the hot burning wood that is constantly stoking the fire. Both must be eliminated before permanent relief can be attained.

Resources to help

Using the whole gamut of resources available such as acupuncture, herbs, nutritional support, sensitivity repatterning and pathogen elimination is a holistic approach to help restore the digestive system to a healthy state. I have worked with many patients who have come to me labeled with one of the above disease processes. Many of these patients are now well, due to this holistic approach. Rebuilding the damaged gut lining is essential to full recovery.

References

Abuhammour, Walid, M.D. "Shigella Infection," eMedicine, Accessed August 7, 2005.
www.emedicine.com/PED/topic2085.htm

"Campylobacter Infections," Division of Bacterial and Mycotic Diseases, Centers for Disease Control and Prevention, Accessed May 9, 2004.
www.cdc.gov/ncidod/dbmd/diseaseinfo/campylobacter_g.htm

Chacon-Cruz, Enrique, M.D. "Intestinal Protozoal Disease," eMedicine, Accessed March 10, 2005.
www.emedicine.com/ped/topic1914.htm

Deadman, Peter and Mazin Al-Khafaji. *A Manual of Acupuncture*. Vista, California: Eastland Press, 1998.

Engstrand, L. "Mycobacterium Paratuberculosis and Crohn's Disease," Department of Clinical Microbiology, University Hospital, Uppsala, Sweden, 2006.
www.ncbi.nlm.nih.gov/entrez/query.fcgi?cmd=Retrieve&db=PubMed&list_uids=8 8671776&dopt=abstract

Frye, Richard E., M.D. "Gastroenteritis, Bacterial," eMedicine, Accessed March 9, 2005.
www.emedicine.com/MED/topic855.htm

Gan, H., Q. Ouyang and H. Bu. "Mycobacterium Paratuberculosis in the Intestine of Patients With Crohn's Disease," Department of Gastroenterology, First Affiliated Hospital, West China University of Medical Sciences, Chengdu, April 1997.

www.ncbi.nlm.nih.gov/entrez/query.fcgi?cmd=Retrieve&db=PubMed&list_uids=1
0374282&dopt=abstract

Goodgame, Richard W., M.D. "Gastroenteritis, Viral," eMedicine, Accessed March 9, 2005.
www.emedicine.com/MED/topic856.htm

Greger, Michael, M.D. "Paratuberculosis and Crohn's Disease: Got Milk," January 2001.

Hiong U Go, Chi, M.D. "Escherichia Coli Infections," eMedicine, Accessed March 9, 2005.
www.emedicine.com/MED/topic734.htm

Kroeger, Hanna. *Parasites, the Enemy Within*, Hanna Kroeger Publications, 1991.

Prantera, C. and M.L. Scribano. "Crohn's Disease: The Case for Bacteria," Division of Gastroenterology, Nuovo Regina Margherita Hospital, Rome, Italy, 2006.
www.ncbi.nlm.nih.gov/entrez/query.fcgi?itool=abstractplus&db=pubmed&cmd=R
etrieve&db=PubMed&list_uids=10379488&dopt=abstract

Ross, Emma. "Some Headaches May Be Linked to Common Germ," *The (Aberdeen, Washington) Daily World*, April 27, 2002.

"Shigellosis," Division of Bacterial and Mycotic Diseases, Centers for Disease Control and Prevention," Accessed June 5, 2004.
www.cdc.gov/ncidod/dbmd/diseaseinfo/shigellosis_g.thm

Snyder Sachs, Jessica. "Are Antibiotics Killing Us?" *Discover*, November 2005.

Stein, Rob. "Mystery Intestinal Bug Striking More Patients," *The Olympian*, December 31, 2005.

Y Ang, Jocelyn, M.D. "Campylobacter Infections," eMedicine, Accessed August 7, 2005.
www.emedicine.com/PED/topic2697.htm

Chapter 28: Neurological Disorders

The categories of these disorders are numerous, so I will try to touch on the most common ones. Neuropathy is a general term that covers many symptoms and generally means some type of nerve disorder. The main disorders are: multiple sclerosis, restless leg syndrome, bipolar disorder, meningitis, arachnitis, Parkinson's disease, neuralgia, neuritis and Lou Gehrig's disease. Some of the common symptoms are shooting pain, numbness, weakness, depression, anxiety, decreased hand coordination, decreased sensations in one or both extremities, and a prickling or tingling feeling in the extremities.

Neurological conditions

Neurological conditions can be caused by several factors. A common cause can be a simple spinal misalignment either in the brachial or lumbar plexus (neurological pathways). A chiropractor can usually take care of this fairly easily. Spinal misalignment can also be caused from over-contracted muscles. The scalene muscles in the neck and even the pectoralis minor muscles in the chest can become tight and pinch off the brachial plexus causing numbness in the hands. A tight piriformis muscle in the gluteal area can also cause numbness and possibly shooting pain that could affect the legs and feet. A well-trained massage or physical therapist can release those muscles. Sometimes a combination of massage and chiropractic works best to correct spinal misalignment, so this should be considered first.

The next cause of numbness and shooting pain, which is probably more common than you think, is pathogens that have entered the spinal cord or are sitting along a nerve plexus, or within a dural tube (meningeal tissue) and/or the brain itself. The dural tube is a wrapping around the spinal cord that serves as a protection against injury. It is also referred to as meningeal tissue, which extends up into the skull and surrounds the brain, connecting to the cranial bones. It is part of the cranial sacral system. This type of connective tissue has three layers: the dura mater (outer and toughest layer), arachnoid (middle layer) and pia mater (delicate membrane enclosing the spinal cord and brain). This tissue is laced with nerves and blood vessels. Any disturbance within this tissue from pathogens, heavy metals, toxins or injuries will influence spinal and neurological function. Sometimes a cranial sacral therapist can help to unblock kinks in this tissue. There are thousands of these therapists within the United States. They usually are licensed as massage or physical therapists or osteopathic physicians with special training in this method. I would be careful to choose one who is well trained and practices this technique on a regular basis. You do not want someone just starting out, since technique, training and experience equal better results.

The role of pathogens

The types of pathogens that can invade the spinal cord and surrounding dural tube can vary. We have all heard of meningitis, which occurs when a pathogen enters the spinal cord and/or brain causing an acute or a chronic low-grade inflammation. The acute symptoms are fever and a severe headache that will not go away. This can be life threatening. However, a lingering pathogen can enter the brain, spinal cord or meninges without causing such an acute episode. The symptoms and severity may vary depending on what type of bug or bugs are present, their numbers in population and the location of tissue that they are invading. For instance, you may have pathogens in the meningeal tissue and nerve roots at cervical one of your spinal cord. The pathogens may cause headaches and facial pain because those specific nerve roots affect these areas. Another example might be a pathogenic invasion occurring at cervical seven/thoracic one. This might cause numbness in the hands, or a subtle feeling of not being able to grip something like you are used to. If these invaders grow in numbers and enter other surrounding tissue and get into the cerebral spinal fluid, which is the highway to the brain, then possibly other more severe symptoms may arise. This can cause an acute episode of meningitis to occur as the brain starts to swell. If the same problem exists in the lumbar spine and is affecting the lumbar plexus, the symptoms might be numbness in the legs with low-back pain and/or possible shooting pains down the back of the leg.

A chiropractor may believe the spine is subluxated (a partial dislocation) in this area and attempt to align it, thinking that a good adjustment will solve the discomfort. She may not realize that there is another factor, out of the chiropractic scope of thinking, which is causing the patient's discomfort. To eliminate the problem, the chiropractor would need a pathogen extractor, which is not handed out in any chiropractic school that I am aware of, or any other school for that matter. The symptoms may never go away, and both patient and chiropractor are left confused and frustrated. A few patients have told me that chiropractic, massage or acupuncture does not work, because it did not work for them. These therapies all work for what they were intended to do. The cause of the disease has to fall into the category of what they were designed to address. If subluxation is the primary cause, then a chiropractic adjustment would have worked. If the neck and gluteal muscles were over contracted, then massage therapy or acupuncture would have worked. A carpenter does not use a hammer to cut wood. Why would you expect anyone with a medical specialty to repair something for which they were not trained to do? You would not think of asking your plumber to make an electrical repair for you, would you?

Multiple sclerosis is a degenerative condition that is usually caused by the immune system attacking various pathogens as they sit in or on the spinal cord and its related structures. The myelin sheath is the outer covering of nerve tissue, so guess what gets damaged first? The delicate myelin sheath. It carries the nerve conduction and transmission of signals. The decrease of signal transmission becomes the effect that leads to paralysis, which is then called multiple sclerosis. Once the myelin sheath is destroyed, there is very little, if any, hope of recovery because nerve tissue does not repair itself. People with these conditions need to address the root cause of the problem. Otherwise, they may end up in a wheelchair, and then it is too late.

Paralysis and numbness may also come from a part of the brain that controls movement, such as the premotor cortex, cerebellum or brain stem. Anywhere that damage is being done to an area containing nuclei (nerve cell bodies), which control specific motor functions, will cause a degradation of whatever function those nuclei control. Autopsies have shown that those with Parkinson's disease have damage to the base of the brain. This is where the key dopa receptors are located. A lingering pathogen in the medulla oblongata may affect breathing, because a major portion of the nuclei in the medulla oblongata control breathing. Generally, any lingering pathogen in any area of the brain could damage delicate brain and nerve structures, thereby causing a symptom in another part of the body, as the brain controls everything. It is the general in command of the body.

A damaged general gives faulty instructions. Hitler had Parkinson's disease, and it worsened as World War II raged on. Some of his decisions toward the end of the war were erratic, not coming from a sound mind. His condition greatly contributed to the United States and Britain winning the war. He can be seen in footage with a trembling arm and hand. See Chapter 20: Mycobacteria.

Specific pathogens

Here are the pertinent pathogens that are fond of entering neurological tissue. First and foremost is our friend, Mr. Lyme disease, a spirochete called *Borrelia burgdorferi*. This bug can cause so many neurological symptoms that it is hard to pinpoint one or two. It can enter the spinal cord and go up to the brain. It has the ability, along with another spirochete called *Neisseria*, to coil and thrust itself into and through tissue. The interesting thing about the Lyme-causing bug, *Borrelia burgdorferi*, is that most people who have it can never recall being bitten by a tick. Many will test negative for it in a blood test.

Years ago my dog was infected with ticks while hiking in Central California. I pulled more than twenty ticks off him. Six months later he became very sick, as these spirochetes invaded his digestive system. He could not hold down any food, so I had to have him put to sleep. Had I known the reality of what was happening, he could have lived several more years, as he was an extremely healthy dog to that point. The vet thought it was cancer, and so did I. It was not long after that when I learned about Lyme disease.

This bug can be passed on in several ways. The first possibility of transmission is through the womb, if mom is the pathogenic carrier. Another possibility is entry from the male in the sperm itself. The third is to actually be bitten by a tick. Lastly, transmission can be made through a blood transfusion. It can invade many places in the body outside of the central nervous system. Spirochetes can sit in the digestive system, lungs and any organ, for that matter.

A patient of mine who was a public speaker had a constant eye twitch for many years. He could not control it and had tried everything conventional medicine could offer. Even acupuncture had failed. Once his immune system was able to remove the lingering pathogens, then the symptomatic eye twitch was greatly reduced. Because he had the eye twitch chronically for years, some irreversible neurological damage had already been done. But he was still very pleased with the improvement. In addition, his low-grade depression, which he did not mention to me until later, just seemed to melt away in the process.

Another younger gentleman came to me with an eyebrow twitch. He had seen several medical doctors, including a neurologist, and they had done extensive testing. Their diagnosis was that the cause was unknown, and he would just have to live with it, or take drugs that had some serious side effects. He only had this symptom for a short period prior to seeing me. When his immune system was able to remove the lingering pathogen, then the twitching stopped. He was able to return to normal functioning, as the damage was minimal. Incidentally, his low libido seemed to recover, as well.

Lyme disease not only causes depression, but may also be the underlying cause of spaciness, vertigo, confused thinking, anxiety and panic attacks. Imagine a cluster of spirochetes residing in your brain or nerve tissue causing havoc, as well as producing toxins. Many patients' mental conditions will completely change once the spirochetes are eliminated. I have also seen numbness either greatly reduced or completely disappear once the eviction process was complete. Lyme disease may be one of the fastest growing illnesses in the United States. Much of Lyme disease's symptoms are misdiagnosed due to the diversity of how it manifests symptomatically, the ineffectiveness of present testing methods and the lack of awareness of your health professional (Fletcher, 2001).

Mycoplasma infection can also enter nerve tissue, including the brain and spinal cord, and can stimulate neurological autoimmune types of symptoms. When one of these bad critters gets in the central nervous system, there is no telling what the symptoms might look like. Many symptoms could be similar to Lyme disease. *Mycoplasma incognitus* is always at the top of the mycoplasma list. This pathogen can mimic Lyme disease symptoms if embedded in the brain or spinal cord. Next up is that familiar parasite, *Toxoplasma gondii*. This bug loves the brain and is mentioned in Chapter 31 on Chronic Depression. It is a common bug to have as mothers carry it and pass it on to their children while in utero. It can cause a host of problems besides depression, including foggy thinking, anxiety, irritability, bipolar disorder and schizophrenia, which are common manifestations of this bug. Brain damage in infants is attributed to this parasite (Achenbach, 2005).

Generally, any aggressive bug will cause widespread neurological symptoms and long-term damage if left untreated. These pathogens will constantly irritate your nervous system. They will damage brain tissue, which can lead to numerous types of symptomology, including brain tumors.

A recent patient came to me with chronic headaches that could not be explained by any medical expert she had seen. She had a brain scan that revealed some demyelinated nerve tissue within her brain. Once her immune system was able to remove the specific brain pathogen, then the headaches completely stopped. The pathogen had been sitting in her brain for years causing damage. That is why the brain scan showed demyelinated tissue.

Remember, these bugs cause inflammation in the brain and spinal cord. They can also cause damage and symptoms to peripheral nerves, as well. If, say, a mycoplasma is sitting on the sciatic nerve, you probably will have shooting pain or numbness in that nerve. Since that nerve extends to the foot, then numbness may be involved in the foot and toes of that leg. Inflammation leads to damage, which leads to more symptoms. It is a vicious cycle.

What bugs cause meningitis? Meningitis can be acute and needs to be addressed immediately or you could die. The brain swells with fluid and becomes inflamed in response to the pathogens. Subacute meningitis is not life threatening, but can cause damage over time.

There are numerous bugs that can cause acute or chronic meningitis. The two most common are the bacteria *Streptococcus pneumoniae* and *Neisseria meningitis*. Other bacteria that are less likely to cause meningitis are: *E. coli, group B Streptococcus, Listeria, Klebsiella, Enterobacter, Staphylococcus aureus, Aceinetobacter, Pseudomonas* and *Haemophilus influenzae*. ECHO virus, herpes simplex virus 2, lymphocytic choriomeningitis virus and coxsackievirus usually cause viral meningitis in children. These all have the potential to cause meningitis. Viruses and bacteria tend to cause the more acute forms of meningitis. Mycobacteria and fungi lean toward the more chronic variety because they are slower to develop.

The common fungi that can cause low-grade inflammation in the spinal cord and brain are: *Cryptococcus, Candida albicans, Aspergillus, Histoplasma capsulatum, Blastomyces dermatitidis* and *Coccidioides*. The mycobacteria are: *Mycobacterium tuberculosis, Nocardia* and *Leptospira*. Parasites can also enter the spinal cord and brain. These include: *Naegleria, Rickettsia* and *Schistosoma*. The truth is, any parasite can enter your body and end up in the spinal cord and brain.

The underlying foundation for this process has to do with how the bug enters your body, your current intestinal environment, and any predisposing injuries you may have had to the spinal cord, meningeal tissue and brain. For instance, you may have acquired a mycobacterium by breathing it into your sinus cavities; this area is in close proximity to your brain. Swimmers can pick up certain water parasites that can enter through the ear or mouth. A bacteria or parasite may have been acquired through ingestion at your favorite salad or sushi bar. This bug may have gotten into your intestinal defense system due to intestinal dysbiosis (lack of friendly bacterial environment and damaged intestinal wall) and, eventually, makes its way into your spinal cord. There are so many variances that they are impossible to track in any scientific way. My general rule of thumb applies here as well, "Anything can go anywhere, at anytime."

Toxic material

Anything that the immune system sees as an offender will provoke an attack. For example, a toxic material, such as mercury, has leached itself from your dental fillings into nerve or brain tissues. The immune system will attack it over and over again and cause a constant, low-grade inflammatory condition to persist, which equates to constant low-grade damage to vital tissue. The immune system was not programmed to remove mercury, so it gets confused and keeps attacking it without success. It could also be any heavy metal or toxic substance that was not designed to enter your body.

We do not know how many toxic materials we are now in contact with in our lives on a regular basis. We also have no idea the downside of some of these substances in relationship to our internal environment. Some may cause unseen damage due to sudden or long-term exposure. In this case, they may be a direct irritant to the nervous system that causes long-term immune responses. This can be true for people who have been diagnosed with multiple chemical sensitivity. This condition may have been set off by exposure to a toxic chemical that short-circuited the nervous system. The immune system's function is to seek and destroy, as that is its purpose. Any number of the symptoms mentioned above should be addressed as soon as possible, as permanent damage can take place if left untreated.

Notes

Achenbach, Joel. "Cat Carrier: Your Cat Could Make You Crazy," *National Geographic*, August 2005.

Fletcher, J.D. and Tom Klaber. "Lyme Disease: The Unknown Epidemic," *Alternative Medicine*, May 2001.

References

Andreae-Jones, Sarah, M.B., B.S. "The Inflammatory Nature of Adhesive Arachnoiditis," A.S.A.M. Society, Accessed May 26, 2005. www.arachnoiditis.info/content/the_adhesive_arachnoiditis_syndrome/the_adhesive_ arachnoiditis_syndrome_5.html

Bode, Liv, Detlef E. Detrich, Roman Stoyloff, Hinderk M. Emrich and Hanns Ludwig. "Amantadine and Human Borna Disease Virus in Vitro and in Vivo in an Infected Patient With Bipolar Disorder," *The Lancet*, January 18, 1997.

"Coxsackie Viruses," Kids Health for Parents, Accessed June 5, 2004. kidshealth.org/parent/infections/bacterial_viral/coxsackie.html

Deadman, Peter and Mazin Al-Khafaji. *A Manual of Acupuncture*. Vista, California: Eastland Press, 1998.

Fallon, Brian A., M.D., M.P.H., and Jenifer A. Nields, M.D. "Lyme Disease: A Neuropsychiatric Illness," *The American Journal of Psychiatry*, Vol. 151, Issue 11, 1994.

Howenstine, James, M.D. "New Ideas About the Cause, Spread and Therapy of Lyme Disease," *Townsend Letter for Doctors and Patients*, July 2004.

King, John W., M.D. "Cryptococcosis," eMedicine, Accessed March 3, 2005. www.emedicine.com/MED/topic482.htm

Kumar, Ashir, M.D. "Meningitis, Bacterial," eMedicine, Accessed June 8, 2005. www.emedicine.com/ped/topic198.htm

"Nocardia Infection," MedlinePlus, U.S. National Library of Medicine, National Institutes of Health, Accessed June 5, 2004. www.nlm.nih.gov/medlineplus/ency/article/000679.htm

Nadalo, Lennard, M.D. "Brain, Abscess," eMedicine, Accessed June 8, 2005. www.emedicine.com/radio/topic91.htm

"Rheumatoid Arthritis and Multiple Sclerosis—The Cause May Be in the Blood," *Alternative Medicine Digest*, Issue No. 18, 1996.

Richt, Jurgen A., Islode Pfeuffer, Matthias Christ, Knute Frese, Karl Betcher and Sibylle Herzog. "Borna Disease Virus Infection in Animals and Humans," *Emerging Infectious Diseases*, July-September 1997.

Strick, Frank. "Micro-Organisms and Mental Illness," *Nexus New Times*, July-August 2004.

"Varieties," Meningitis Foundation of America, Accessed October 4, 2002. www.musa.org/varieties.htm

Chapter 29: Lyme Spectrum Illnesses

Lyme disease is a chronic infection that that is caused by a tick bite, as well as other transmission avenues. Chronic Lyme disease and its co-infections are epidemic in the United States, as well as many other countries. The Centers for Disease Control and Prevention (CDC) used to report 30,000 new cases of Lyme disease a year in the United States (Harris, July 2015). However, the agency recently revised its estimate to 300,000 per year.

Daniel A. Kinderleher, M.D., internist, stated on the Today Show that 1.8 million cases of existing Lyme disease reported by the CDC had been under reported by at least ten times. Actually, there are 18 million cases (Walker, August 6, 2007). This was prior to 2007. In the United Kingdom, Lyme disease has increased 90 percent since 2006 (Rosner, July 2010). The world's leading Lyme pediatric specialist Charles Ray Jones, M.D., medical director of Pediatric/Adolescent Medicine and Lyme Disease Clinic, said that everyone is at risk including newborns. Of the 5,000 children he has treated, 240 have been born with the disease. A leading authority in integrative medicine said there are very few symptoms where Lyme disease should not be considered, since a quarter of the population in the United States may be affected. "More than 50 percent of all ill people may have Lyme contributing to their condition," said W. Lee Cowden, M.D., cardiologist, clinical nutritionist and internist.

The B31 strain in the United States and Europe is genetically identical. This indicates a migration of the organism in recent years. The B31 strain is the most common in the Northeast part of the United States. This strain is most virulent of them all. The farther you travel from the Northeast, the strains become more diverse. This could affect both the symptoms patients may be experiencing and their test results. Not all strains infect humans, some just cause the rash. There are at least four strains that can get beyond the skin and cause internal damage. These invasive strains have much different capabilities. There has been a resurgence of interest in the topic of Lyme disease due to the increasing numbers of people being infected worldwide and a wealth of new updated information that has come out in the last few years, indicating that Lyme disease is much more than just an acute illness (Rosner, July 2010). There is a big discrepancy on how this condition manifests into long-term symptoms. Traditional medicine and the CDC take the approach that Lyme disease is only contracted through a tick bite and is curable with a short course of antibiotics. Progressive Lyme literate doctors and a growing number of health care providers have a completely different understanding of Lyme disease. This illness is a long-term chronic infection that can cause a myriad of serious symptoms. Many people may be infected and have no symptoms, while others will become quite ill. The next section examines these differences at a much deeper level.

Difference in perspectives

First of all, the traditional medical system does not seem to understand or acknowledge chronic low-grade systemic infection as the cause of many of their labeled diseases. This means that either the infection is there in full force, or it is nonexistent. An allopathic doctor's education and understanding of chronic infection in the body is very limited. Within the traditional medical mindset, Lyme diseases can only be contracted by a tick bite. The bite will show a bull's-eye skin response and a positive Western blot test result will reveal the infection. A three-week course of antibiotics will cure the infection and we will all live happy ever after, just like in the Wizard of Oz. Unfortunately, this illusion only happens in traditional Western medicine and fictional tales. Many unsuspecting patients will buy this misguided information because of their own lack of knowledge. When a Lyme sufferer presents typical Lyme symptoms, most doctors, as well as alternative medicine health providers, do not understand that a chronic Lyme infection may be causing or at least contributing to the symptoms being presented. Doctors are so conditioned to see and treat just the symptoms that an infection is never on their radar, or prescription pad.

Secondly, it is difficult to get a positive Western blot result due to the lack of updated information about the testing method.

Thirdly, there is much misguided information on how Lyme disease can be acquired. Even if a doctor suspects it could be Lyme disease, which is rare, the Western blot test will usually not show the infection. Then the patient is scratching his or her head because the tests come back negative, and the doctors assure them that they do not have Lyme disease. Many times they are told that the symptoms are in their head, which in reality is one of the primary places that the spirochete *Borrelia burgdorferi* is hanging out. Many natural medicine doctors may look for a vitamin or blood deficiency, or claim it is a detox issue, while a doctor of acupuncture may see it as a qi, blood or yin deficiency. We need to all wake up and smell the Lyme disease. I believe there has been much progress in educating doctors recently. As time goes on, more and more are increasingly becoming Lyme aware.

Pretend for a moment that you actually had a positive Western blot test. Following a three-week course of antibiotics, the *Borrelia burgdorferi* infection is supposed to be gone (Stringfellow, July 13, 2016). However in many cases, within a short period of time, a multitude of symptoms slowly begin to manifest. These symptoms mimic Lyme disease. The patient is then given a new diagnosis called Post-treatment Lyme Syndrome (Smith, July 2010). According to this new disease label, you no longer have Lyme disease because the antibiotics had killed it. Instead, you now have a syndrome caused by the previous Lyme infection. With Post-treatment Lyme Syndrome, drugs that treat the numerous symptoms are once again the standard protocol.

This is another example of how traditional medicine continues to hang disease labels on people with no known cause or cure. More importantly, this is a very poor understanding of what is actually taking place. A deeper look into *Borrelia burgdorferi* will show what makes it tick.

The great imposter

These potent strains have the ability to exchange genetic material with each other, which enables them to self-replicate. They can merge with other cells and carry out functions, which benefit both the host cell and themselves. They have a negatively charged outer surface protein with an altered three-dimensional surface structure. This enables them to change surface shape and internal structures instantly with millions of potential variations. *Borrelia burgdorferi* has the ability to learn how the innate immune system functions and to use this knowledge to evade immune responses. *Borrelia burgdorferi* contains more than 100 variable proteins. These proteins can change their expression on their outer surfaces appearing to be one thing and then becoming something totally different. Plasmids are much like the DNA of the cell. They hold the information for survival. They are incorporated into the cell and govern its functions. A plasmid can encode information for a certain type of antibiotic or antibody and store this within its own information system. This and much more encoded information is used to preserve the species when a threat is eminent. It is always one step ahead of the immune system, much like in a real-life battle where the enemy has captured the blueprint of the next attack and is just waiting so they can move their troops in position to ambush the attack. Some soldiers may die in the process, but others will remain and encode that information for the next attack. Plasmids use this information to change shape and form. *Borrelia burgdorferi* contains twenty-one plasmids, a much higher number compared to other bacteria. This enables it to store unlimited information, and it has the ability to out maneuver the natural immune system, as well as every type of weapon cast upon it. This includes antibiotics, herbal and other therapies. This is why these types of treatments must be rotated on a regular basis for best results. Between its cell wall and outer membrane is an extension of flagella. This helps it navigate through denser parts of the body such as connective tissue and hard to reach areas that the immune system, antibiotics and antimicrobials cannot reach. Molecular mimicry is another weapon *Borrelia burgdorferi* possesses, which allows it to alter its surface protein molecules to look like proteins of normal cells and tissue, thereby confusing the immune system into thinking that it is one and the same. The immune cells see *Borrelia burgdorferi* as itself, at times hindering the attack, or in some cases causing more damage. The immune system attacks its own healthy tissue. This is what is referred to as an autoimmune disease. The body is attacking itself, but for a good reason. Nothing in the body is by accident. Every action causes a reaction.

There also is a strong indication that *Borrelia burgdorferi* releases a toxin (Bradford, February/March 2006). This would be similar to the enemy in battle releasing a nerve gas in order to hinder your defenses. These toxins or poisons are referred to as a mycotoxin or neurotoxin. This is another way in which *Borrelia burgdorferi* causes so much continual damage and toxic overload, increasing symptoms, pain and tissue deterioration. Knowing how *Borrelia burgdorferi* is built and how it functions once it enters the body leads to a deeper understanding of why a three-week course of antibiotics cannot totally kill it. There is even much misunderstanding in the alternative medical community, which also fails to understand chronic Lyme disease. Ticks can carry a smorgasbord of disease-causing agents that enter the body simultaneous with *Borrelia burgdorferi*.

Borrelia burgdorferi is the cause of Lyme disease. It is part of the spirochete family, along with many other spirochete strains including syphilis. It is the most invasive and aggressive of all the strains. Other pathogenic strains that may have been carried by the tick are known as co-infectants (Forsgren, July 2015). These are *Ehrlichia*, *Rickettsia*, also called Rocky Mountain spotted fever, *Babesia* and *Bartonella*. A tick can carry several of these strains along with various mycoplasma strains, leaving the human hosts with years of potential suffering ahead. There are also several different strains of *Borrelia burgdorferi* depending on which part of the country people were infected in. The Northeast strain seems to be the most aggressive one. A deeper look into the physiology of *Borrelia burgdorferi* will show why it is so aggressive and hard to kill.

Borrelia burgdorferi in many ways has some similar characteristics that both mycoplasma and HIV possess. Spirochetes and mycoplasmas are both intracellular, which means they can hide inside other cells and tissue, especially red and white blood cells. They are both pleomorphic, which allows them to change shapes instantly. They also have no cell wall, which allows for their stealth capabilities. They can change from one form to another instantaneously with unlimited cell structure and surface variations. The immune system has a hard time recognizing cell wall deficient microbes. When *Borrelia burgdorferi* changes to a cyst or bleb form (round), it can reside in a dormant state for years, able to withstand antibiotic therapy. It is the antibiotics that drive *Borrelia burgdorferi* into this form (Overbye, July 2015). This resting state is just waiting for the right opportunity to come out and invade the body. The spirochete form is the active form that travels through the system reproducing. This allows it to rapidly spread throughout the body. Spheroblasts or L-forms are the most sophisticated types. These lack a cell membrane, so they can travel about and evade immune detection, making it difficult for the immune system to lock onto them. This also affects the testing results, because their antibodies are not detected by current testing standards. All these forms produce protective biofilms and can invade any tissue in the body, especially the brain, spinal cord, organs, glands and joints. As previously mentioned, they create various toxic byproducts called mycotoxins and neurotoxins that play havoc within the central nervous system (brain and spinal cord). They can overload the lymphatic system and, over time, deteriorate organ and glandular functioning, specifically the kidneys, spleen and adrenals. *Borrelia burgdorferi* is the gate opener for other less invasive pathogenic forms to take hold and contribute to the overall picture. Much like HIV, you do not die from HIV, but from the accumulation of all opportunistic infections that eventually take the whole system down. Candida overgrowth, bacterial and parasitic infection, mold sensitivities, nutritional deficiencies, hormonal imbalances, glandular and organ deterioration, lymphatic overload, impaired detoxification pathways and joint, brain and neurological damage all encompass the overall chronic Lyme disease package.

Neurotoxins

Some Lyme disease experts think that neurotoxins produced by the *Borrelia burgdorferi* itself are a large contributing factor to the symptoms caused by these pathogenic microorganisms. A neurotoxin is a poison that acts specifically on nerve cells. They are absorbed by the nerve ending and then travel inside the neuron to the cell body. The toxins cause the nerve cell to malfunction. They distort the messages of the nerves to any part of the body. The toxins are closely similar to *Clostridium botulinum*. They then can greatly affect the release and availability of key neurotransmitters, particularly dopamine, serotonin and acetylcholine. With diminished neurotransmitter activity and the gradual buildup of these toxins within key structures of the central nervous system, mental processing will become very slow. Symptoms of brain fatigue, memory issues, depression, inability to focus, balance problems, rigidity, muscle pain and general lethargy become the norm. People forget what it was like to feel happy and have interest in life and work. The mental energy to take on life with rigor is long gone. Many people are currently on one or more drugs for depression, but this treatment ignores the cause and allows these toxins to continue to build up within the body and brain. This is why the success rate for treating depression with prescription drugs is so poor. The huge increase in psychiatric prescriptions the last few years has risen in proportion to the rise in Lyme disease, vaccinations and Alzheimer's disease. Vaccines, mercury fillings, aluminum and other heavy metals can also cause similar types of toxins to form in the brain.

Biofilms

Biofilms are another area that has gained a lot of attention in association with Lyme disease lately. Biofilms seem to create another protection mechanism that *Borrelia burgdorferi* employs in its arsenal of tools (Kenner, July 2015). This has to do with multi-pathogenic communities that build a biofilm fortress around themselves for protection and the preservation within this housing colony. This substance looks like slime under a microscope and is produced by the pathogens themselves. These microbes use the slime substance as a protective shelter. The materials used for construction within this living matrix may include certain glycoproteins, calcium and magnesium. This becomes the home for various species, which could include *Borrelia burgdorferi*, several different strains of spirochetes, as well as mycoplasma, bacteria and other pathogenic organisms. These organisms have been observed leaving and entering the biofilm colony. The biofilms have many internal structures that assist the transport of water, toxins and nutrients. These colonies have coordinated cell to cell communication called quorum sensing. This way of communicating allows for coordinated movements within the colony. The colonies can set up shop in almost any area, but prefer the more remote and protected areas such as the joints, brain, soft tissue and old injury sites.

Symptomology

One of the most common symptoms of a Lyme carrier is the continual deterioration of brain functioning. Memory and cognitive thought processes are usually lacking due to the chronic brain inflammation and subsequent release of neurotoxins that inhibit neurotransmitter activity and brain function. Serotonin and dopamine pathways are hampered by these toxins. This is why antidepressant therapy focusing on neurotransmitters has such a low success rate. This long-term process eventually leads to progressive damage in the brain. The question then arises: Does Lyme disease cause Alzheimer's disease? The plaque formation that accumulates in the nerve tissues, neurons and blood vessels of the brain is characteristic of what is seen in Alzheimer's disease. This plaque is an effect of the chronic neural inflammation that is caused by the long-term presence of one or more pathogens that inhabit the brain.

Kris Kristofferson, the actor and songwriter, was diagnosed with Alzheimer's, chronic fatigue and fibromyalgia only to learn that Lyme disease was the cause of these symptoms. His cover story in *Closer* magazine is entitled "Miracle Recovery…From Alzheimer's Diagnosis" (*Closer*, August 1, 2016). This is an account of his journey in finding a Lyme aware doctor whom at first did the standard Western blot test which came back negative for Lyme disease. The doctor then had more advanced lab testing done, which confirmed the chronic Lyme infection. Kristofferson is doing much better because he is being treated for the cause of the symptoms. He stopped taking his medications for Alzheimer's and fibromyalgia once his treatment for Lyme disease began. Alec Baldwin, Ben Stiller and Parker Posey also are part of the article as they are also being treated for Lyme disease. These are real people who looked above the symptomology and disease labels for the true cause.

Other symptoms that accompany this ongoing brain inflammation include sleep disorders, usually waking up at night and not being able to get back to sleep. Other brain issues include forgetfulness, irritability, foggy thinking, posterior neck pain, occipital (back of head) headaches, depression, tinnitus, anger, mood swings and brain fog. Chronic joint pain and inflammation that can travel from one area to another is a typical symptom that *Borrelia burgdorferi* causes. The shoulder injury that never healed. The chronic back and neck pain that just will not go away. The deteriorated spinal discs that were never injured. Peripheral nervous system effects include numbness, tingling and shooting pains (Forsgren, July 2010). Skin symptoms include itching, psoriasis, eczema, hair loss or graying, facial twitching and scalp tenderness. Visual disorders include eye deterioration, macular degeneration, cataracts, floaters and eye twitching. Other general effects include high blood pressure, fluid imbalances, heart irregularities and gastric reflux. Lack of energy is usually a big part of the picture as well, including the chronic fatigue that has become part of a person's everyday survival mode. They forget what it was like to have energy and enthusiasm. The body's energy reserves are feeling the constant drain that is going on within. Gradual weakening of the vital organs and glands is occurring.

Borrelia burgdorferi can also thrive in the genital-urinary system and can cause kidney deterioration, high blood pressure, interstitial cystitis (chronic bladder inflammation), vaginal, cervix and prostate inflammation and even cancer. The Lyme pathogen can invade any part of the body and cause progressive damage. It has a tendency to invade the lumbar sacral plexus, a collection of cell bodies and spinal nerves that innervate the lower extremities. Restless leg syndrome is usually caused from *Borrelia burgdorferi* and its presence within the lumbar sacral plexus. Once it invades the plexus, there is a continual hyper stimulation that causes the involuntary movement of limbs. Why it happens at night has to do with the rise of inflammation within the body as the day and evening progress. The more heat, the more stimulation. This also has to do with the nervous system not able to expel excess energy at night while at rest. Secondary complications of *Borrelia burgdorferi* infection include hormonal dysfunction, methylation detoxification pathway defects that affect the liver, kidney and skin, lymphatic overload and intestinal dysbiosis (imbalanced intestinal bacteria). Much of the workload ends up being done by the liver, kidneys, skin and lymph system. That is key to gradual organ degradation.

The co-infectants

Co-infectants are other pathogens that are transferred with the tick bite to its host (humans). The common co-infectants are:

Bartonella is an intracellular parasite that causes an infection in the circulatory system (red blood cells and its vessels), as well as the bone marrow (Forsgren, July 2015). This parasite can cause a host of cardiovascular symptoms such as endocarditis and myocarditis (inflammation of the heart wall). It can adhere to the inner lining of the blood vessels (endothelium) including the veins and heart valves causing damage. This parasite can disrupt blood flow with restricted microcirculation throughout the vascular system, especially the smaller blood vessels in the brain and other areas such as the extremities and teeth. Blood filled sacs in the liver are possible along with Inflammation of the neural retina and optic nerve. This can be a causative factor in heart attack, heart weakness, plaque buildup, blood thickness and vascular coagulation. Typical neurological symptoms such as pin point or dull headaches, severe anxiety, mental and emotional imbalances, rage, depression, muscle and joint pain and skin disorders. Lab testing for *Bartonella* is not accurate as false negatives are common, meaning the infection is present, but it is not able to be detected with current testing methods (Forsgren, July 2015). It has a low population and hangs out in the blood vessels, red blood cells and cardiovascular tissues and seldom flows freely in the bloodstream. Recent research has identified eight or so species, but potentially many more have not been as yet discovered. *Bartonella* is usually carried by the tick and released into the bloodstream or by being bitten by fleas or from cat scratches.

Babesia is one of the most common co-infectants that resides inside the red blood cells of its host (Schaller, July 2015). Two different strains exist: *Babesia microti* and *Babesia duncani*. The symptoms can be numerous and severe including fatigue, migraine headaches, night sweats, nightmares, cough, shortness of breath, heart arrhythmia, low red blood cell count, weight fluctuations, clotting problems and neurological symptoms (Harris, July 2010).

Ehrlichia is a gram-negative bacteria. Ehrlichiosis is a term for the disease that is acquired through its transmission from a tick bite by the lonestar tick. Muscle pain, fatigue, low white blood cell count, bleeding issues, breathing difficulties, fevers, chills, fatigue, rash, headache, confusion, nausea, vomiting and diarrhea are the most common symptoms. This organism infects the white blood cells and will circulate in the bloodstream. Blood transfusions are a common way of acquiring it.

Rickettsia is a gram-negative, highly pleomorphic bacteria. The classification of Rickettsia into three groups (spotted fever, typhus and scrub typhus) was based on serology. This grouping has since been confirmed by DNA sequencing. All three of these contain pathogens that can cause a myriad of disease like symptoms. They tend to invade the inner lining of organs causing weakness and progressive organ dysfunction.

Anaplasma is carried by the black-legged tick. It is found in the Northeastern and Eastern United States. The symptoms are similar to rickettsiosis.

Not much information is available on the risk of passing the above co-infectants during sexual intercourse. However, transfusions would be a much easier way to receive them and possibly through womb transfer. Various forms of mycoplasma are easily transferable, much like spirochetes (Lyme disease).

Mycoplasma: See Chapter 21: Mycoplasmas.

The disease labels

Because chronic *Borrelia burgdorferi* infestation functions as a lingering pathogen that may be causing or contributing to symptoms or effects, these symptoms are placed into a labeled disease category that the medical system and insurance companies relate to. They include attention deficit disorder, autism, multiple sclerosis, arthritis, ankylosing spondylitis, chronic fatigue syndrome, Lou Gehrig's disease, fibromyalgia, Alzheimer's disease, Parkinson's disease, migraine headaches and psychiatric labeled disorders of all kinds including anxiety, depression and panic attacks. Other symptoms are restless leg syndrome, tinnitus, bursitis, Meniere's disease, tendonitis, vaginitis, prostatitis, lupus, heart disease, diabetes, cancer, Sjogren's syndrome, eczema, dermatitis, hair loss and facial neuralgia. The list goes on and on. You name it and there is a medical disease label for whatever symptoms that may be manifesting from the missed or undiagnosed ongoing Lyme infection. It is right under their nose but most doctors just cannot seem to smell it. This is not to say that *Borrelia burgdorferi* is causing every disease label. But in many cases it may be at least part of the overall picture. *Borrelia burgdorferi*, its co-infectants and mycoplasma are usually the driving force behind the barrage of unrelated symptoms that baffles the traditional medical mindset as well as most alternative medicine practitioners.

Children and Lyme disease

There seems to be a strong association between Lyme disease, autism and attention-deficit/hyperactivity disorder (ADHD). Since Lyme can be acquired in vitro during pregnancy, the symptoms of the above two labeled diseases and Lyme are closely associated. The sharp rise in the last few years of both autism and ADHD has followed the steep rise in the diagnosis of Lyme. If more adults are shown to be carriers, then naturally their offspring will have a good chance of acquiring it. This has to be part of why there are so many kids showing signs and symptoms of Lyme disease, relabeled into autism, ADHD, depression, slow learner or other disorders. The most common ways children contract Lyme disease is by transference in the womb from mom and breastfeeding.

There is a much higher chance to contract Lyme disease if you have lived in a high tick area of the United States. These include the Northeast (especially Connecticut, New York, the New England area and Pennsylvania), Virginia, Kentucky, Ohio, Missouri, the entire upper Midwest, the South, Northern and Central California (which includes the Sierra Nevada mountain range), Idaho, Montana, Eastern Oregon and Washington and Southern Oregon. Again, you do not need to be bitten by a tick to contract the illness.

In 2000, my dog was bitten by twenty-one ticks near San Luis Obispo on the Central California coast. He mysteriously got very ill and died six months later. The vet did not know the cause, but the more I learned about Lyme disease over the next few years, the more I realized what had made him so ill. Had we not taken that walk near all the oak trees, he would have avoided the tick bites. My girlfriend and I stayed on the path, but Buddy explored off in the brush and that is where the twenty-one ticks attached to him. We did not realize he had been bitten until we got back to

Seattle and gave him a bath. Buddy would have lived many more years as he was in fine health.

The Lyme disease spectrum

New forms of *Borrelia* are being discovered all the time. *Borrelli miyamotoi* and *Borrelia myonii* are two potentially dangerous forms that were only discovered in the past few years. *Borrelia mylophora* is probably the least known. These three are very common and within the *Borrelia* (Lyme) spectrum. I call it a spectrum because most people are not carrying just one strain, but multiple strains along with one or more mycoplasma. These three strains mentioned above are not yet being tested for, even in the best labs. Therefore, getting a negative result for *Borrelia burgdorferi* does not rule out that people are carrying one or more of the other potent strains mentioned above. *Borrelia mylophora* is the worst of these three, as it attaches itself to the brain and spinal cord. These top four are implicated in multiple sclerosis, restless leg syndrome, Lou Gehrig's, Parkinson's and a host of other neurological symptoms and disorders. Ways in which you can contract these have expanded and include bites from mosquitoes, fleas and bed bugs and transfusions, sexual intercourse and the womb (Walker, August 6, 2007). *Borrelia* and syphilis are both in the spirochete family. We know the latter is considered a sexually transmitted disease. A recent small-scale study testing sexual partners' sperm and vaginal fluid confirmed the same pathogenic strains of *Borrelia* are likely being passed during sexual intercourse.

The diagnosis testing process

The testing methods for *Borrelia burgdorferi* have been unfortunately subjective and lack certainty. The reason most people are not diagnosed with Lyme disease as the cause of these above symptoms has to do with how Lyme symptoms and their effects are not recognized by the consulting health professionals. Many infected people are never tested for what is actually causing their symptoms. Others may be infected but have little or no symptoms because their immune system was able to control it. Allopathic medicine uses the Western blot test or the enzyme-linked immunosorbent assay to determine if the infection is present. This type of testing in most cases comes up negative, even though many times an infection is present. Then the patient is told that they do not have the infection, therefore the symptoms must be due to an unknown cause, or possibly a genetic defect. The patient then is left with the only option available, leading them down the same old drug path by once again chasing symptoms around the body. This is the same approach on every illness, which always ignores the cause. My research leads me to believe the Western blot

Lyme's test used exclusively for testing *Borrelia burgdorferi* will unfortunately give many patients who are carrying it a false or negative reading, when the patient is positive. There are much more accurate forms of testing that are designed to show the Lyme infection, if it is truly present. Millions of Americans are now infected with one or more varieties of spirochetes without ever gotten bit by a tick. They go from doctor to doctor, trying to find answers for their symptoms. The few lucky ones find a Lyme aware doctor. When one is trying to get a true and accurate test result, several labs are available that offer a comprehensive testing menu that encompasses testing for the co-infections as well, especially *Bartonella, Babesia, Ehrlichia* and mycoplasma.

The CDC sets the guidelines requiring that those tested have both IgG and IgM responses to a particular number of bands. IgG responds to a chronic long-term infection and IgM indicates a recent active infection. Many times the IgG will come up negative because over time the immune system may get tired and the white blood cell production may go down. The Western blot uses only a few highly reactive strains of *Borrelia burgdorferi* and ignores other ones. Some of the other strains may be less sensitive to this type of testing. Testing can also be swayed by *Borrelia* itself affecting IgG and IgM levels by suppressing them. It is known that *Borrelia burgdorferi* over time can reduce the number of white blood cells by killing off a percentage of them, which can eventually show up as a depressed immune response on blood tests. Then there is the cell wall deficient form, which most current testing methods lack the ability to be able to detect. Most labs only test for one to three strains when in reality there are dozens of strains. Many labs cannot duplicate the result from one lab to another. It appears that Western blot testing for *Borrelia burgdorferi* is at best hit and miss. Here are a few of the competent testing facilities:

- IGeneX: Palo Alto, California, comprehensive Lyme and co-infective testing.
- LabCorps: Burlington, North Carolina, CD-57 panel, which evaluates natural killer cell receptors that are depressed in chronic Lyme disease.
- FryLab: Phoenix, Arizona area, comprehensive Lyme and other related pathogenic testing.

Antibiotics and their role

Aside from the initial three-week course of antibiotics, some Lyme literate doctors are using long-term, low-grade antibiotics as their primary treatment modality. This treatment can reduce the overall spirochete numbers. However, other complications can compromise the overall situation. First of all, *Borrelia burgdorferi* has various forms, the spirochete form, the cell wall deficient form and the cyst/round form. Antibiotics are effective against the active spirochete forms, but not the cyst/round doormat form, which allows *Borrelia burgdorferi* to hibernate inside white blood cells and joint tissue. Then it is able to reappear in the spirochete form, once the antibiotic therapy has stopped. This is why most people who choose this route are on endless antibiotic regimes, having to repeat this over and over again. The other important disadvantage to antibiotic therapy is that it compromises the intestinal integrity by causing intestinal yeast overgrowth (*Candida albicans*) and dysbiosis (gut flora imbalances). See Chapter 13: Antibiotics.

The cover-up

Many educated Lyme patients and doctors think that the CDC is purposely down playing the real numbers of chronic Lyme disease sufferers for several reasons. This is an exploding disease of epidemic proportions. You would think that the CDC would want to protect the public. After all, that is its job, right? The amount of money that a misdiagnosed patient might spend over the course of a disease by ignoring the cause and treating symptoms would be in the tens of thousands of dollars compared to knowing what is causing the symptoms in the first place. Low-grade antibiotic therapy is much less expensive. You add to that the potential illness that can escalate by allowing the *Borrelia burgdorferi* to fester untreated while you are chasing around symptoms. This nontreatment of the real cause can develop into escalating health issues down the road. A potential Lyme patient could cost our health care system half million or more in long-term symptom control care and surgeries over a lifetime. This is another example of why national health care costs are going up astronomically. What motive could the CDC have in trying to hide the true numbers by preventing hundreds of thousands of patients annually from knowing the true cause of their illness? A Western blot Lyme test at best only shows a small percentage of the actual true numbers. Why is donor blood not being screened? That has already started with the Zika virus, which has only a small number cases reported compared to millions with Lyme disease. Many Lyme literate health professionals know that a Lyme diagnosis takes into account many factors that include symptoms, history of where you were born and have lived, number of sexual partners, transfusions and, of course, tick bites. Lab testing can be used as part of the overall picture, but the practitioner should not rely on those tests solely. This is called a clinical diagnosis. Because *Borrelia*, mycoplasma and the co-infectants are so difficult to test for, multiple tests may be needed to determine their presence.

Going forward

I see Lyme disease playing a big role in the future of illness, especially Alzheimer's disease. Not identifying it as the causative agent in a multitude of modern disease processes will surely drive up health care costs, let alone all the suffering that will occur. It is scary to think that one little tick bite can cause such long-term suffering, or that one sexual partner may be the donor, the gift that keeps giving. Many individuals in the United States are infected and do not even know it. Their method of transmission may not have been a tick bite. We are conditioned to believe that we have to call a set of symptoms a labeled disease in order to identify it. Our thinking about chronic spirochete infestation needs a huge awareness leap. This needs to start with the health professionals such as naturopathic physicians and licensed acupuncturists. Unfortunately, there are restrictions placed on medical doctors to see and diagnose Lyme disease for what it is, a potentially long-term debilitating illness, instead of a set of symptoms on a prescription pad. Acupuncture and naturopathic medicine schools need drastic changes in their education, as most students leave these institutions with little or no knowledge of this epidemic. They need to learn how to recognize Lyme disease in a patient and how to be able to effectively treat it. Updated testing methods need to be the norm so it can be properly identified. We need to become more aware of what is right under our nose. We need to see a set of symptoms as an effect of the cause that is progressively worsening and poisoning the body. Prescribing only temporary relief for symptoms (drug or herbal medicine) without addressing the cause is not what is best for the patient. Being aware of the potential causes should be what we all should strive for, not just temporary symptom relief.

Notes

Bradford, Robert W. and Henry W. Allen. "Biochemistry of Lyme Disease," *Townsend Letter*, February/March 2006.

Forsgren, Scott. "Saving Our Children: Evaluation and Management of Pediatric Tick-Borne Diseases," *Townsend Letter*, July 2010.

Forsgren, Scott. "Unraveling the Mystery of Bartonellosis," *Townsend Letter*, July 2015.

Harris, Steven, M.D. Excerpt from *Insights Into Lyme Disease Treatment: 13 Lyme-Literate Health Care Practitioners Share Their Healing Strategies*, "Chapter 1: Chronic Lyme Disease Treatment," *Townsend Letter*, July 2010.

Harris, Steven, M.D., and Mischa Grieder, N.D. Interview with Nancy Faass, *Townsend Letter*, July 2015.

Kenner, Dan, Ph.D., L.Ac. "Multifactorial Approaches to Lyme Infection," *Townsend Letter*, July 2015.

"Kris Kristofferson's Miracle Recovery…From Alzheimer's Diagnosis," *Closer*, August 1, 2016.

Overbye, Bjorn Johan, M.D. "Lyme Disease: A Microscopist's Search for an Antibiotic-Free Solution," *Townsend Letter*, July 2015.

Rosner, Bryan. "Lyme Disease: An American Problem or Worldwide Plague?" *Townsend Letter*, July 2010.

Schaller, James, M.D., and Kimberly Mountjoy. "Advanced 2015 Babesia Care: Profound Testing Defects and Preventing Disability and Death," *Townsend Letter*, July 2015.

Smith, Hal. "Connecticut's Antitrust Action Against IDSA's Lyme Guidelines: Medical Guidelines Development Demands Scientific Procedures," *Townsend Letter*, July 2010.

Stringfellow, Barry. "Visiting Physician Sheds New Light on Lyme Disease," *Martha's Vineyard Times*, July 13, 2016.

Walker, Morton, D.P.M. "What Makes Lyme Disease Tick and How Samento Eliminates It," The Medical Journalist Report of Innovative Biologics, August 6, 2007.

Chapter 30: Alzheimer's Disease

Alzheimer's disease is the disease of our time that is predicted to escalate exponentially with each passing year. The economic impact on the American health care system will be even more severe. Presently one in every five Medicare dollars is being spent on Alzheimer's disease. Six million people in the United States currently have either Alzheimer's or Parkinson's disease. In 2015, $226 billion dollars was spent on Alzheimer's and dementia related illnesses. This is a huge part of what is already an economically overburdened medical system. Why this disease has come about during our time has to do with many factors that were not present during past generations. The factors behind this disease are both diverse and constant, which combined cause long-term neurological degeneration to occur within the brain. This process is currently impacting many Americans to some degree without them knowing it.

The Alzheimer's diseaseprocess

Alzheimer's, which is brain inflammation, is a silent slow-moving killer that presents itself in progressive symptoms over time. Most people are not aware of the ongoing degenerative process in their own brains. Current and future generations unfortunately will be impacted even more by this evolving disease process. This is another medical disease label that seems to have appeared out of nowhere, much like many others before it. Alzheimer's, like all the others, has no known cause or cure by medical professionals. The best medical minds are once again baffled by what could be destroying so many people's lives.

It makes more sense to call this brain inflammation and understand what causes it, instead of another medical disease label without a cause or cure like so many before it. Inflammation almost always plays a key role in every disease process, and it could not be truer in this case. Alzheimer's disease is the result of years of chronic inflammation in the brain. This inflammation causes amyloid beta plaque buildup and damage to the sensitive nerve fibers and blood vessels that keep the brain firing properly. When they do an autopsy on an Alzheimer's patient, their brain is filled with this type of plaque formation and damaged nerve tissue. This substance only forms when chronic inflammation is present over a period of time. It is much like how inflammation causes plaque to form on artery walls, or how joint cartilage is progressively damaged over time. Without inflammation, heart disease, arthritis, Alzheimer's and most of the chronic illnesses cannot occur. The symptoms and structural changes seen in Alzheimer's disease is the same as chronic inflammation in the brain. Inflammation is the never the underlying cause, as it is always the effect of the cause, or the secondary factor which then causes the damage. How do people know they have the early signs of Alzheimer's disease?

Early symptoms

Poor memory and gradual cognitive loss is associated with a person who has dementia or Alzheimer's disease. However, going back in time in an Alzheimer's patient's life, their steps can be retraced like a movie in reverse as the beginning of this process starts to unfold. How this happens is not a mystery but an explainable process. This can start as early as conception. However, in most cases early warning signs usually start to appear in one's thirties or forties. These symptoms could have included foggy or slow thinking, sleep disturbances, falling asleep but waking up soon after, forgetting things you used to remember, lack of mental stamina, loss of interest for life, a feeling of heat in the head, especially at night, night sweats, irritability and decreased mental buffering, which is when an outside stimulus easily triggers emotional reactions such as fear or anger. Subtle changes occur at first in terms of the above symptoms, but as the years pass, the symptoms get progressively worse. This could be considered the early and middle stages of brain/neural inflammation or Alzheimer's disease. The poor memory and loss of cognitive thinking can evolve to total loss of brain function and eventual death as the last stage of this process. The disease may start very early in life beginning in the womb, and continue for decades until the apparent symptoms actually manifest.

Many factors cause the gradual brain deterioration seen in Alzheimer's disease. Among them are the following:

Pathogenic invasion

The first and most common cause of brain deterioration is pathogenic invasion of the central nervous system (the brain and spinal cord). Many people can have these organisms living within them and never know it because the inflammation is at a subacute level. The medical mindset of infections as being either non-existent or full bore is narrow, outdated, black-and-white thinking. The Centers for Disease Control and Prevention recently released an update on Lyme disease saying that the problem is grossly underestimated. There are more than 300,000 known new cases a year, according to the CDC. This is up 90 percent from their previous estimate of 30,000 new cases a year. *Borrelia burgdorferi*, a spirochete that causes Lyme disease, as well as several other closely related spirochete forms, and *Mycoplasma incognitus* are the likely suspects setting up shop within the brain and spinal cord causing a chronic low-grade inflammatory process. These are common pathogenic forms that can be sexually transmitted and coexist within much of the population. *Borrelia burgdorferi* and other spirochetes, along with *Mycoplasma incognitus* and certain parasites and viruses, such as the herpes virus 1, 2, 6 and 8 can live in the brain from conception as it is sometimes acquired in the womb. Spirochetes have the ability to coil like a snake and inject themselves into the spinal cord, reaching the cerebrospinal fluid. Once in the cerebrospinal fluid, they can travel into the brain and start their replication process and life cycle. Brain tissue is a safe and healthy environment for these organisms to flourish in, as the immune system has limited abilities in this area. See Chapter 28: Neurological Disorders and Chapter 29: Lyme Spectrum Disease for more complete explanations.

Vaccinations

Another factor is vaccinations. Most vaccinations can have aluminum, cadmium, mercury and formaldehyde in each dose. During my childhood, I received only a few vaccinations. However, most children are now being vaccinated more than twenty times. Mercury and aluminum are easily absorbed by the brain. Adults who follow doctor's orders by getting their yearly flu, shingles and other vaccinations can also be at increased risk. The more people are vaccinated the higher the chance is for these toxic metals to accumulate in the brain. There is enough evidence that shows these metals have an affinity for neurological tissue. They can adhere to this tissue and become a focal point for the immune system to attack. This ongoing process stimulates the inflammatory process, thus causing long-term neural inflammation and brain deterioration. Mercury is a known toxin that if injected into the bloodstream can attach itself to the brain. In populations that do not vaccinate, there are no cases of attention deficit spectrum disorder (ADSD). A clear example of what a vaccination can do to the brain in an elderly person was my mom. When she was ninety-two and still mentally and physically healthy, she went to a doctor for a checkup without telling me. That evening I was at her house for dinner, and it was apparent that she was not herself. She complained of severe mental fogginess and felt terribly depressed. I inquired what she had done that day, and she confessed she had gone to the doctor for a simple checkup and the doctor insisted she get two vaccinations, supposedly for the flu. The symptoms slowly faded over the next few weeks, but two years later a brain tumor formed. There is no solid proof that these shots caused the tumor, but my mom lived an extremely clean lifestyle and was so healthy. There was no possible reason that a brain tumor would grow without something causing it. Mercury lodged in the brain causes persistent immune stimulation that can form into a tumor in some cases. I believe those vaccinations were a causative factor in her brain cancer. The documentary *Vaxxed: From Cover-Up to Catastrophe* should be watched by all as it exposes the vaccine industry and the measles, mumps and rubella (MMR) vaccine and its relationship to neurological symptomology.

Dental work

Dental work, specifically fillings that are composed of mercury and other toxic metals that can slowly leach out and end up poisoning the delicate brain and nerve structures, is another cause of brain deterioration. in dental fillings, which was standard protocol for years, is still being used by some dentists. Mercury can easily leak into nearby tissues and be absorbed by the brain. Because fillings are permanent, these toxins are constantly interacting with the immune system as they are released every time you chew. Many dentists have mercury free alternatives. The debate on whether mercury used in fillings is harmful has been going on for years. The American Dental Association still supports the use of mercury in fillings.

Low cholesterol

An even more interesting factor in brain decline is low cholesterol in the body. Lowering cholesterol has been a huge agenda for the medical system, which has been pushing low-fat diets and cholesterol-lowering drugs. Low cholesterol makes the brain venerable to damage by reducing the substance the brain needs to protect itself. Cholesterol serves as an insulator of the brain, protecting it from damage from free radicals and inflammation. The idea that people need to keep cholesterol under 200 to prevent cardiovascular disease is not true. Low cholesterol slowly destroys the body and brain tissue. With lower cholesterol, damage from the various sources is greatly accelerated.

Air pollution

Another cause of brain deterioration is air pollution. Some pollutants can be seen such as car and diesel exhausts and airplane emissions. This is visible air pollution. The chapter on electromagnetic/invisible smog reveals how invisible smog can also slowly damage the brain. This is invisible air pollution. Cell phones should not be put up to the ear, as this process slowly fries the brain. An interesting cover story from *Mother Jones* magazine is called "Does Pollution Cause Dementia?" (Reuben, July/August 2015). This article claims that it is the ultra-fine particles, thirty-six times smaller than a grain of sand containing nitrates, sulphates, ammonia, hydrocarbons and heavy metals, especially aluminum, are some of the key culprits causing dementia. The long-term exposure to these particles is paving the way for brain damage to take place. Some of the other key points from this article are as follows:

The olfactory system

This system of smell is the first to encounter these toxic chemicals. A possible prerequisite to Alzheimer's and Parkinson's disease is the gradual loss of smell. This reveals the slow degenerative process of the olfactory system. As these particles enter the nose, the larger ones are filtered out by the nasal hairs. These particles send messages about the content of what is currently passing through this system. They are then transmitted through the olfactory nerve to your brain. This is why many drug users like to snort drugs as they can get an immediate high. These tiny particles and messages trigger an immediate immune assault as the brain sees it as a foreign enemy. They will slowly accumulate in the brain, causing a long chronic immune assault that damages sensitive tissues over time. The immune system was not designed to be able to remove such particles. This is like having an autoimmune brain disease that keeps the assault up much like multiple sclerosis, rheumatoid arthritis and other autoimmune diseases. If the immune system is attacking any area of the body over a period of time, it does not matter what the source is – pathogenic, toxic metals or allergic reactions. Persistent inflammation will cause more and more damage to occur the longer it is ongoing. The brain is slightly different from other parts of the body because of the delicate nerve structures that it is made of are very slow to regenerate.

Microglia cells

Microglia cells are like patrolling policemen and garbage collectors of the brain all in one. Their job is to be on the lookout for any criminals such as invading microorganisms and toxic metals, as well as any leftover trash called microscopic debris that has invaded the brain. Their weapons are chemical compounds that can be released to kill the invaders. When a pollutant cannot be removed in this manner then these compounds accumulate and start to kill healthy cells that are surrounding the foreign particle or lingering pathogen. The microglial cells mistakenly perceive particles from pollution as foreign invaders such as a heavy metal or pollutant. Constant brain agitation leads to brain deterioration.

Age

People age fifty and older are much more venerable to brain degeneration, according to the latest research. The process is greatly sped up in older adults. This age population is manifesting brain degeneration much faster than younger people with the same exposure load.

Brain trauma

A newly recognized factor in gradual brain deterioration is brain trauma. One single trauma to the brain may cause microscopic brain damage, but repeated traumas will compound the damage. Trauma can be from a difficult birth, such as the use of forceps, sports injuries including one or more concussions, as in professional football and boxing, as well as auto accidents that involve head trauma or injury. Any impact to the brain that causes swelling to occur will cause damage at some level. Repeated trauma seems to greatly increase this damage.

High blood and brain glucose

High insulin levels trigger inflammation. Insulin spikes are a result of high sugar ingestion. This process is outlined in a *Well Being Journal* article called "A Nutritional Approach to Prevent and Heal Alzheimer's and Metabolic Syndrome" by Amy Berger, M.S., NTP (Berger, January/February 2016). Recently, there has been a sharp increase in the awareness and scientific explanation of the causes of Alzheimer's disease. This article comes at it from mostly a nutritional standpoint, focusing on diet and specific nutritional suggestions. There is some good science in this article that explains how diet and lifestyle choices over time can help to prevent brain damage from happening and the physiological effects of diet on the brain. It helps explain an important piece of the puzzle.

Some of the key points of the article pinpoint specific regions in the brain that affect memory and learning. A reduction in the rate in which the brain uses glucose occurs in these venerable areas. This process can start in younger years before any external signs present themselves. Metabolic syndrome is a host of markers that can show an improper utilization of carbohydrates. Plaque formation in the brain can be much greater due higher levels of insulin. Remember that increased insulin levels increase inflammation, which is the true cause of cardiovascular disease as well. See Chapter 25: Cardiovascular Disease. Plague formation is a direct response to inflammation. If certain key brain regions are not using glucose properly then that could cause damage over time. Insulin spikes followed by low blood sugar are the culprits. This pro-inflammatory rebound effect has many other negative side effects as well. Key brain regions become deficient during the rebound effect, and they are literally being starved for fuel. Whole grain foods, proper oils and daily exercise are a basis for a healthy lifestyle. This keeps the insulin spikes at a minimum.

Metabolic syndrome is a term that has been used for several years to describe the improper utilization of carbohydrates. When overconsumption of refined carbohydrates is combined with the continual stress of modern life and lack of sleep as well as little physical activity, it leads to a breakdown in the body's and brain's ability to process carbohydrates and other fuels (Berger, January/February 2016). High glucose spikes are a key part of this picture. This article also makes a strong argument for the connection between Alzheimer's and type 2 diabetes. This connection is consistent with my chapter on diabetes, which describes the real cause of it. The relationship between the brain and diabetes has to do with cell wall and brain tissue health. Both must use healthy fats to function properly. The brain as mentioned earlier uses cholesterol as an insulator, protector and basis for proper nerve transmission. Each cell wall is composed of a bi-lipid layer. Lipid means fat and bi means double. Low cholesterol or fat in the body robs both the brain and each of the body's cell walls causing poor functioning and eventually progressive damage to these areas. The chapter on diabetes explains how this slow deterioration of the cell wall leads to diabetes and poor cell assimilation of nutrients. If they cannot get through a damaged cell wall, insulin, nutrients and glucose accumulate outside the cell, because the doors are locked. The chapter on cholesterol explains the importance of having sufficient amounts of healthy cholesterol for these vital areas to draw from.

The glymphatic system

Although the brain weighs about three pounds, it consumes 20 to 25 percent of the body's energy (Nedergaard, March 2016). The brain also eliminates a quarter of an ounce of worn-out proteins that must be replaced daily. The *Scientific American* article contains information from the author's research and some is slightly speculative, but overall it is informative. It describes the glymphatic system, which acts like the lymphatic system to drain away waste products and is managed by brain cells called glia cells. Waste products and dead proteins that are not flushed out of the brain can accumulation and turn into protein clumps, or aggregates, according to researchers. These aggregates are consistent with the amyloid beta plaque formation seen in Alzheimer's disease. They can impede the transmission of electrical and chemical signals in the brain and cause irreparable damage. This cleansing system of the brain is much more active at night while at sleep.

Sleep disturbances affect how this system operates. It is believed that poor sleep will cause malfunctions in clearing the protein aggregates away. This difference can decide who eventually gets an Alzheimer's diagnosis and who does not. Astrocytes are a type of glia cells in the brain and spinal cord. They have extensions called end feet that surround every vein, capillary and artery in these areas of the nervous system. The end feet open to the perivascular space—an exterior part of the blood vessel—that is a passageway for fluids surrounding these blood vessels. Astrocytes play a key role in the movement of fluids in this area. During the sleep process, the glymphatic system is most active clearing away toxins and other metabolic substances that interfere with nerve transmission and help to prevent a buildup of this material, which leads to the aggregate plaque formation that is seen with Alzheimer's disease. Poor sleep and other factors reduce the amount of activity with this cleansing system. Therefore, the longer and deeper you sleep could greatly affect your body's ability to cleanse itself of these poisons. The problem is that many people with brain pathogens will have poor sleep due to the heat and toxins produced daily.

Accumulation

Many scientists now believe that it is not one thing, but a combination of many factors that are part of our life, such as the food we eat, air we breathe and water we drink, which causes Alzheimer's. In the early 1900s, people had to go to a phone booth to make a call. When phones were made available for the home, they had a cord. People had no computers and WiFis. They inhaled clean air free of toxic metals and damaging particles. Their food was naturally grown and life was much slower and simpler. People are breathing in, ingesting things and passing microbial organisms between them through sexual intercourse and womb transmission that are slowly destroying their brains and bodies.

Money

Money also is a factor in brain deterioration. I met a man last year whose wife was dying from Alzheimer's disease. I asked him what he was doing to help her. I suggested coconut oil as a start. Research on this oil has been impressive and many people that have taken it in adequate amounts on a daily basis have seen improvement. He told me that he took his wife to the top Alzheimer's research center/clinic in Scottsdale, Arizona, and was told by the head of the center that coconut oil did not have any benefit. The sad thing is this elderly man thought that answer was the truth. I doubt if the clinic or the doctor that saw a study did any research on it. There would be little profit in the clinic promoting coconut oil rather than high-cost prescription drugs.

The medical system has no answers for Alzheimer's disease like so many before it. The money is never in the cure, but in the promise of a cure, which perpetuates the disease. Future drugs for Alzheimer's will bring in billions per year. It will greatly raise insurance premiums and add to the burden on Medicare and ultimately people's pocket books. Billions will be raised to supposedly find a cure and the result will be much like the cure for cancer, arthritis and all the other labeled diseases, always just out of reach. This has been a trademark for how the medical system profits from sickness. None of the drugs developed will ever address the cause. The cure will be just another medical illusion. Despite the efforts of many in this country to reverse the progressive downward spiral of the planet's overall health, big business continues to pull the strings and control the overall picture.

People have been programmed by the medical establishment to believe that dementia and poor health are a natural part of the aging process so people feel accepting when it happens to them. Poor us, how did we get this horrible disease, they ask their doctors? The answer is always the same; no one knows exactly what causes it, but there are drugs to slow the process or improve the symptoms. Mind control in medicine is a very powerful tincture that perpetuates so much within American culture.

New Alzheimer's factors

Many of the factors causing brain deterioration were non-existent twenty years ago. This is why so many people are experiencing brain decline after they reach age forty. It takes many years before the brain starts to show signs of the disease process that may have started at birth, or early in life. Worldwide death from lung disorders such as lung cancer, chronic obstructive lung disease and lower respiratory infection total more than 700,000 and heart disease and stroke almost three million (Reuben, July/August 2015). This shows that what people inhale has to end up somewhere in the body and the tissues that are in the closest proximity to the nose and mouth are the lungs, heart and brain.

Air pollution either visible or invisible affects all of us. The amount of exposure, plus the total time of exposure equals trauma to the brain. Even weather reports can give an indicator of both the coarse particles and ultrafine particles in the air that day. I grew up in Los Angeles during the 1960s and remember many smog alert days.

This was before unleaded gas was required. A dark cloud would hang over the city and would cause people to cough. School was canceled on some of these days.

Reversing chronic brain inflammation

This degenerative process needs to be caught as early as possible. Removing or reducing the pathogenic load not only in the brain, but also in the entire body is beneficial as any inflammation will rise upward and affect the head. Heat in the head either produced locally or systemically will be a component of this process. The more heat, the greater the chance for progressive damage to occur over time. The longer people are exposed to electric smog or multiple environmental pollutants, especially aluminum, mercury and cadmium, increases the chance that they will get Alzheimer's disease. Protection of the brain is critical. Reducing systemic and localized inflammation and healthy cholesterol over 200, along with lots of good fats and the correct antioxidants, will serve as protection against further damage and may start reversing the damage. The higher the healthy fat intake the better off people will be as fat serves as neurological insulation. Coconut and olive oil along with organic butter will support the brain as low-fat diets and cholesterol lowering drugs are a set up for rapid brain degeneration and early Alzheimer's onset. People must lower their bodies' inflammation, especially in the gut and brain. Testing for C-reactive protein and an oxidation stress test are the two most valuable tools for indicators of present inflammation levels and ongoing oxidative damage. Detoxification of heavy metals using chelating agents to reduce the load is important. Chlorella, cilantro and liposomal glutathione used together on a daily basis will help this process. Liposomal curcumin and liposomal vitamin C along with coconut oil will help reduce the inflammation in the brain and body.

Conclusion

Enough science has revealed why Alzheimer's is becoming so common. The only ones who fail to acknowledge the numerous causes are medical experts who ignore the real science because it never leads down the golden pathway. This pathway is lined with green, the type you can always bank on. People have to do their own research as this can lead to the knowledge that we are all seeking in our own health care.

Notes

Berger, Amy. MS, NTP. "A Nutritional Approach to Prevent and Heal Alzheimer's and Metabolic Syndrome," *Well Being Journal*, January/February 2016.

Nedergaard, Maiken and Stephen A. Goldman. "The Brain's Waste-Disposal System May be Enlisted to Treat Alzheimer's and Other Brain Illnesses," *Scientific American*, March 2016.

Reuben, Aaron. "Does Air Pollution Cause Dementia?" *Mother Jones*, July/August 2015.

Chapter 31: Chronic Depression

Millions of people live daily with depression without much hope. Many have turned to prescription drugs, and in some cases have found help. But others are still plagued by this lifeless existence and have nowhere to turn; drugs do not seem to be the answer for them. Depression, like other symptoms in the body, has a cause. Depression can come from an acute emotional episode such as a spouse dying or from a physiological defect within the body.

Physiological causes

The most common cause of chronic depression is brain chemistry problems involving key neurotransmitters. Serotonin is the brain chemical that allows us to be naturally happy. When the body lacks serotonin, then depression, foggy thinking and sleep problems coexist. Serotonin is the most important brain chemical. Small imbalances can make a huge difference in how we feel. Most drugs for depression focus on increasing the uptake of serotonin. However, side effects can sometimes be as detrimental as the original depression itself.

How is serotonin formed in the brain? The foundation for building serotonin starts with vitamin B complex. Insufficient amounts of this vitamin complex, especially B_6, can lead to a serotonin deficiency. B_6 is a precursor for serotonin, which means that any problems with malabsorption (inadequate absorption of the vitamin or nutrient in the intestinal tract) of this nutrient will cause a deficiency. This deficiency is the first foundational problem that will affect serotonin production. Next are amino acids. There are a half-dozen key amino acids that, if they are not properly absorbed, can lead to neurological and serotonin problems. They are: GABA, tryptophan, glutamic acid, tyrosine and phenylalanine. The most important are the first two. GABA is a calming amino acid that plays a role in neuroinhibition, which means it helps to calm the nervous system. Tryptophan is a direct precursor or builder of serotonin. Serotonin is a precursor of the hormone melatonin, which also aids in sleep and depression. Deficiencies in any of these will affect neurological function and lead to hyperexcitability of the nervous system. The other amino acids play a lesser role in serotonin production. The final level of problems that can exist involves the production and uptake of serotonin itself. Sensitivity to serotonin can lead to malabsorption. This means that you can be sensitive to your own serotonin as well. I refer to this as an internal reactant or sensitivity. You can also be sensitive to the other precursors that I have mentioned above. This is more common than you think. Any kinks in these three levels can cause a lack of serotonin production and/or uptake with any or all of the above-mentioned symptoms. Sensitivities to common foods such as wheat and corn, as well as food additives, can trigger neurological symptoms such as anxiety, anger, brain fog, irritability and depression and can even mimic multiple sclerosis (MS) symptoms. NutraSweet, a common sugar substitute has been reported to cause MS symptoms, as it is a neurotoxin.

Years ago I suffered from moderate to severe depression. I went the usual route of going to several medical doctors and finally to a few neurologists to see if any of them had the "magic pill" so I could feel well again. They explained that I had a lack of serotonin and that it was just a matter of finding the pill with the least side effects that could help my serotonin levels to normalize. I tried several drugs that all seemed to cause obvious side effects, but did not seem to relieve my depression. In fact, I developed serious cardiovascular side effects from this adventure that went on for years. To this day my cardiovascular system has not totally reversed itself from these side effects. That experiment with allopathic medicine was in the early 1980s.

I next went to a natural medical doctor who prescribed large amounts of tyrosine, phenylalanine and vitamin B complex for three months. I tried this without any improvement. She finally put me on a mild drug called trazodone that would knock me out at night. I did not need this drug because I had no trouble sleeping. My depression was still unchanged after two months on the trazodone. Later on, both tryptophan and melatonin came out on the market, and I put those to the test without any significant changes in my depression. (When I was in my teens, I had bad acne that I successfully treated with tetracycline. The only problem was that I had to be on it continually in order for it to work. I was on it for more than two years. Tetracycline is a commonly prescribed antibiotic that kills bacteria.) I had done what all the experts had told me to do, but still my depression was not any better.

A few years later I had a consultation with a gentleman about macrobiotic foods. I told him of the problems I was having, and he felt I might have something called candida, which I had never heard of. He instructed me to eat only protein and veggies for a few days and see how I felt. To my surprise, by the third day most of my depression and foggy thinking were gone. I then researched the fungus *Candida albicans* and found that the antibiotics I had previously taken had caused *Candida albicans* to grow within my body. This was a major contributor to the depression and several other symptoms I was having. However, I still had what I term, a low-level of foggy thinking/slight depression/irritability pattern. This was different from the candida as it was much milder.

In 1994, I took a course to help people overcome their allergic sensitivities. This treatment was designed to permanently help clear allergic reactions and sensitivities. I did not think I had allergies, but I had several patients who could benefit from this technique if it truly worked. After taking the training I put the work aside for a while and forgot about it. However, I eventually started to treat myself for various nutrients that I was sensitive to. One of the first things I treated myself for was vitamin B complex. I noticed an immediate improvement in energy, mood and thinking within days. It was just starting to get interesting. I had been taking extra B complex for years without really noticing any improvement; however, once I repatterned this nutrient complex, my body started to absorb it, and what a difference. As I repatterned other vitamins my health drastically began to improve. I treated tryptophan and melatonin and noticed how much more clearly my thinking was. Salt was another big item as it was causing my brain fog. It was like layers of blockages were coming off piece by piece. After treating magnesium, my entire body and muscles relaxed even further. My serotonin treatment was incredible. The moment I started the clearing process for serotonin, it was like the last veil was being removed. I could feel this rush of happiness and mental clarity come over me. I had removed the last blockage from my brain and it felt awesome. See Chapter 3: My Story for more information.

What this process taught me was that my body was deficient in B complex, tryptophan and melatonin. This caused me to not have the inherent ability to build the proper foundation for producing serotonin, but even more interesting was that I was allergic to my own brain chemical serotonin as well. The treatments were like turning on switches that had never been previously flipped on before.

The role of pathogens

There is one more common cause of depression that I see in my practice frequently. Certain pathogens, and their toxic byproducts, can get into or affect the brain and spinal cord causing depression. Lyme disease, caused from a tick bite that transmits a spirochete, has a way of entering nerve tissue (Achenbach, August 2005). It can coil and inject itself through nerve tissue into the spinal cord and brain. I believe that this bug can cause so many problems with depression that it is relatively a common causative agent. *Mycoplasma incognitus* is a common neurological pathogen that can reside in the brain and cause a number of mental disorders. *Toxoplasma gondii* is a parasite that has been implicated in brain dysfunction. I had a patient who had an immediate improvement in this area once she eliminated it. Borna disease virus has also been implicated in various brain disorders (Bode, May 23, 2007). *Candida albicans* has the ability to enter the brain and spinal cord. This fungus produces a toxic byproduct called acetaldehyde, which can adversely affect depression and brain function. Any type of pathogen such as a virus, bacteria, parasite, mycoplasma, mycobacteria, fungus or mold, or its byproducts, has the potential to affect the brain. Pathogens irritate nerve tissue, and help to create a chronic low-grade inflammatory process. They also produce toxins that can inhibit neurotransmitter production and assimilation. Lingering pathogens can cause so much damage in neurological tissue, which includes the brain or spinal cord, that if left untreated may cause irreversible damage. For many, these bugs cause a constant low-grade irritation to the nervous system that can manifest as irritability and depression. When these pathogens are removed, neurological functioning can return to normal and symptoms usually will improve.

Depression is an effect that can drastically improve once the sources of it are unraveled. Many times there is a combination of the above in the puzzle. You must clear out all the pathogens and allergic/sensitivities that are affecting brain and neurological function. Only then can you begin to understand what has been keeping you from your right to natural happiness.

Notes

Achenbach, Joel. "Cat Carrier: Your Cat Could Make You Crazy," *National Geographic*, August 2005.

Bode, L. and H. Ludwig. "Borna Disease Virus Infection, a Human Mental-Health Risk," Neurotransmitter.net, Accessed May 23, 2007. www.neurotransmitter.net/bornavirus.html

References

Bode, Liv, Detlef E. Detrich, Roman Stoyloff, Hinderk M. Emrich and Hanns Ludwig, "Amantadine and Human Borna Disease Virus in Vitro and in Vivo in an Infected Patient with Bipolar Disorder," *The Lancet*, January 18, 1997.

Fallon, Brian A., M.D., M.P.H., and Jenifer A. Nields, M.D. "Lyme Disease: A Neuropsychiatric Illness," *The American Journal of Psychiatry*, Vol. 151, Issue 11, 1994.

Fletcher, J.D. and Tom Klaber. "Lyme Disease: The Unknown Epidemic," *Alternative Medicine*, May 2001.

Howenstine, James, M.D. "New Ideas About the Cause, Spread and Therapy of Lyme Disease," *Townsend Letter for Doctors and Patients*, July 2004.

Richt, Jurgen A., Islode Pfeuffer, Matthias Christ, Knute Frese, Karl Betcher and Sibylle Herzog. "Borna Disease Virus Infection in Animals and Humans," *Emerging Infectious Diseases*, July-September 1997.

Strick, Frank. "Micro-Organisms and Mental Illness," *Nexus New Times*, July-August 2004.

Chapter 32: Respiratory Disorders

Disorders of the respiratory tract include asthma, pneumonia, chronic obstructive pulmonary disease, bronchitis, respiratory distress disorder and pulmonary edema. These all refer to a variance in the type of effect that has manifested. None of these labels tells us what causes it or how to fix it.

The disorders

Asthma has been around since the Model T. Asthma means that the bronchial tubes are closing off due to inflammation and fluid buildup. Inhalers are the standard treatment for asthma, which can alleviate the symptoms. It is important that if you cannot breathe you need something to open up the airways fast, and inhalers do a good job. It is, however, a symptomatic approach to a deeper problem.

Pneumonia and pulmonary edema are very similar conditions that mean too much mucus is being produced in the thoracic cavity, which reduces the size of lung capacity. This excess fluid also may be produced within the lung itself. Chronic obstructive pulmonary disease means the lungs are not functioning too well, and we do not know what is causing it.

Bronchitis means chronic inflammation of the bronchial tubes. Inflammation causes swelling and heat.

Underlying causes

This section provides information on the underlying causes of various respiratory illnesses, so we can begin to understand how these disorders are developed.

Asthma is known to be triggered by allergies. This is true because the lungs are open to the external environment. This means that any inhaled particles may trigger an allergic reaction, which can cause an acute inflammatory process to take place in the bronchial tubes. These tubes then produce mucus as a protective mechanism. The mucus becomes thick, which restricts the ability of the bronchial tubes to allow the free flow of air. The bronchial tubes can start to spasm in response to the above factors. The most common causes of allergic asthma are attributed to external allergies such as dust, molds, pollens, weeds, trees, etc. These are substances that we breathe in. Reaction to them can start to close off the air passageways and subsequent breathing. Asthma may also be attributed to childhood emotional issues, which may be triggered by certain emotionally charged situations.

Asthma may also be of a pathogenic origin, or pathogens may be at least a co-factor. For example, a lingering pathogen such as *Mycoplasma pneumoniae* may be hanging out in the bronchials. This bug creates a low-grade localized inflammatory process in these breathing tubes. Then add some external allergies such as dust and pollen to the fire. This will create more inflammation and mucus, and you now have a labeled disease called asthma. When the body is able to rid itself of both the lingering pathogens and the offending allergies, then inflammation is reduced or eliminated, and a respiratory dysfunction is no longer present. The labeling of asthma is an effect of this underlying pattern.

In 2006, researchers at the Washington University School of Medicine in St. Louis, Missouri, said that preliminary studies have shown that almost 50 percent of people who experience asthma symptoms have a chronic airway infection that they are not aware of. "It may be that some asthmatics can't get their symptoms under control because low-level respiratory infection is causing inflammation that won't respond to typical asthma treatment," said Mario Castro, M.D., professor of medicine, Division of Pulmonary and Critical Care Medicine. The research was part of a nationwide study on asthma that was sponsored by the National Heart, Lung and Blood Institute of the National Institutes of Health (Ericson, May 9, 2006).

Asthma also has an antibiotic connection as well. In March of 2006, new research published in the March issue of CHEST, the peer-reviewed journal of the American College of Chest Physicians, showed that children under age one who were treated with an antibiotic were twice as likely as untreated children to develop asthma in childhood. In addition, the repeated use of antibiotics in infants appeared to further increase the risk in developing asthma. Lead author of this study, Carlo Marra, Pharma D, Ph.D., University of British Columbia, Vancouver, B.C., Canada, said, "Our overall results show that treatment with at least one antibiotic as an infant appears to be associated with the development of childhood asthma." The coauthor Fawziah Marra, M.D., University of British Columbia, said, "The majority of upper respiratory infections and bronchitis is viral, for which antibiotics are ineffective."

Henry Ford Hospital in Detroit, Michigan, also concluded in their study in October 2003 that antibiotic use in children was linked to higher risks for allergies and asthma. Christine Cole Johnson, Ph.D., the study's lead author and senior research epidemiologist for Henry Ford's Department of Biostatistics and Research Epidemiology theorized that the use of antibiotics may affect the gastrointestinal tract and alter the development of the child's immune system.

I find bronchitis to be caused usually by lingering pathogens. These pathogens sit in these tubes and create inflammation as the immune system is constantly attacking them. The attacks contribute to the inflammatory process by releasing many chemicals that support the inflammation process. Chronic bronchitis can cause a nagging dry cough that can go on and on. Respiratory syncytialvirus (RSV) is the usual culprit. Once it has embedded itself in the mucosal lining, the immune system may fail to remove it. Have you ever met someone who has a constant dry cough, which just lingers for months? They may be the unwilling host for RSV. Other pathogens can also join in and linger throughout the respiratory system. Many of these include bacteria such as *Staphylococcus, Streptococcus, Pseudomonas*, as well as *Mycoplasma pneumoniae*. Common cold viruses such as adenovirus, ECHO virus and coronavirus may linger as well. Molds and fungi can also invade and create havoc. *Histoplasma* is a common respiratory mold that can gradually take over the lungs and cause any of the above symptoms.

Streptococcus pneumoniae, Chlamydia pneumoniae, Mycoplasma pneumoniae, Haemophilus influenzae, Klebsiella pneumoniae and *Staphylococcus aureus* can cause pneumonia. Lingering pathogens and allergies are the main culprits in all of this. I had a seventy-five-year-old patient who had been diagnosed at one time or another for most of the above syndromes. She was on five or six drugs and could hardly walk across the room. She had been using the drugs since she was a child. She had been a nurse most of her life. The labeling of the syndrome, and the symptomatic treatments she had been receiving, did nothing to treat the cause of her illness. The drugs were a Band-Aid at best. Her body was so weak from all the years of drugs and several surgeries that it was an uphill battle to get her well.

Medical experts claim there is no cure for asthma. A better choice of words might be that there is no cure for asthma if you continue to treat it with what allopathic medicine has to offer. It is such a shame, because so many people who live with asthma and other lung ailments could truly get well by seeking other options.

I watched a TV commercial about a popular asthma medication. It clearly stated that there is no cure for asthma, but claimed that this medication would help the symptoms. Some people are vulnerable and easily influenced to believe the commercial programming. If you asked someone who saw the commercial, but had no other prior knowledge of asthma, they would be more than likely to remember these words; "There is no cure for asthma." It is a subtle, but a very powerful way of saying the traditional medical establishment has all the answers. The only option you are offered is to take these drugs on a daily basis in order to treat the symptoms.

In June 2006, national headlines showcased a woman who had severe asthma for one-and-a-half years. She had a lung biopsy, which showed that *Mycoplasma pneumoniae* was found in the tissue sample. She was put on antibiotics and improved drastically. The National Institute of Health awarded the National Jewish Medical and Research Center seven and a half million dollars to see if a bacterium is the culprit underlying asthma. I could have told them that for a lot less money, as I have seen this correlation in my own practice for years. The problem in these researchers' faulty reasoning is that it is not just that one bug that is causing asthma. There may be several bugs that could be possible participants in this process (Fong, June 8, 2006).

In Chinese medicine, asthma is referred to as lung qi deficiency. This is a very treatable and curable condition if you understand what causes it and know how to treat it.

Alternative medicine options

Alternative medicine offers many options for treating respiratory disorders. Acupuncture and herbs can be effective in clearing out the heat and mucus from the lungs and bronchial tubes, as well as strengthening the lungs and supporting the immune system. See Chapter 2: Energy Medicine for more information. Energy medicine can be effective in addressing some of the underlying causes of respiratory disorders, which are usually the lingering pathogens and environmental sensitivities. There are also other nutritional substances and homeopathic formulas that can help support the lungs and immune function. This synergistic approach may be the long-term solution people are looking for.

Notes

Ericson, Gwen. "New Study Challenges Guideline Against the Use of Antibiotics for Asthma," Washington University School of Medicine, May 9, 2006. www.mednews.wustl.edu/news/page/normal/7186.html

Fong, Tillie. "National Jewish [Medical and Research Center] to Hunt for Bacteria-Asthma Link," *Rocky Mountain News,* June 8, 2006.

References

"Antibiotic Use in Infants May Double Asthma Risk," PR Newswire, March 13, 2006. www.prnewswire.com/cgi-bin/stories.pl?ACCT=104&STORY=/www/story/03-13-1281024

Auge, Karen. "Blame It on Bacteria: Germ May Be Asthma Culprit," *The Denver Post,* June 8, 2006.

Brochert, Adam, M.D. "Klebsiella: One Potentially Nasty Bacteria," PersonalMD, Accessed March 3, 2005.
www.personalmd.com/news/klebsiella_102299.shtml

Deadman, Peter and Mazin Al-Khafaji. *A Manual of Acupuncture*. Vista, California: Eastland Press, 1998.

Dittmer, Christine D., M.D. "Bronchitis, Acute and Chronic," eMedicine, Accessed March 4, 2005.
www.emedicine.com/PED/topic288.htm

Harley, William B., M.D. "Mycobacterium Avium Intracellular," eMedicine, Accessed March 3, 2005.
www.emedicine.com/MED/topic1532.htm

"Histoplasmosis," The Lung Association, Accessed March 4, 2005.
www.lung.ca/diseases/histoplasmosis.html

Kaufmann, Doug. *The Fungus Link: An Introduction to Fungal Disease Including the Initial Phase Diet*, Rockwall, Texas: Media Trition Inc., 2000.

Kaufmann, Doug. *The Fungus Link: Volume 2, Tracking the Cause*. Rockwall, Texas: Media Trition Inc., 2003.

King, John W., M.D. "Cryptococcosis," eMedicine, Accessed March 3, 2005.
www.emedicine.com/MED/topic482.htm

Koirala, Janak, M.D. "Mycobacterium Kansasii," eMedicine, March 3, 2005.
www.emedicine.com/MED/topic1537.htm

Krilov, Leonard R., M.D. "Respiratory Syncytial Virus Infection," eMedicine, Accessed March 4, 2005.
www.emedicine.com/PED/topic2706.htm

Ojcius, David M., Toni Darville and Patrick M. Bavoil. "Can Chlamydia Be Stopped?" *Scientific American*, May 2005.

Paulson, Tom. "Antibiotics Prompt Bacteria 'Walls,'" *The Olympian,* August 25, 2005.

Qarah, Samer, M.D. "Pseudomonas Aeruginosa Infections," eMedicine, Accessed March 3, 2005.
www.emedicine.com/MED/topic1934.htm

Sharma, Sat, M.D. "Pneumonia, Bacterial," eMedicine, Accessed March 3, 2005.
www.emedicine.com/MED/topic1852.htm

Stephenson, Joan, Ph.D. "Studies Suggest a Darker Side of 'Benign' Microbes," *Journal of the American Medical Association*, Vol. 278, No. 23, December 17, 1997.

Umeh, Obiamiwe, M.B.B.S. "Klebsiella Infections," eMedicine, Accessed March 14, 2005.
 www.emedicine.com/MED/topic1237.htm

Chapter 33: Chronic Sinusitis

Sinusitis is an inflammation of the sinus cavities, which causes excess mucous production. The mucous is produced as a protective device to prevent damage to the mucosal lining of the nasal cavities. The mucus production then is not the cause, but an effect of the inflammation. The inflammation is not the cause either, because something has to cause the inflammation.

A common problem

Sinusitis is a very common problem that seems to go on and on in some people despite medical intervention. I have worked for years with chronic sinus sufferers who have had long-term inflammation in the sinus cavities, and, for the most part, have been very successful in treating it. This process has revealed to me that the bacterium *Staphylococcus aureus* is the number one cause of chronic sinus conditions.

Causes of sinusitis

Staphylococcus aureus is a common bacterium that has been strengthened by the overuse of antibiotics, which has caused it to mutate and become resistant to further antibiotic therapy. It will survive in the mucous membranes and become a cell wall deficient strain in response to antibiotic therapy. This strain will start to regrow once the antibiotic cycle is over. It has been labeled as a superbug and given a proper title, named *methicillin-resistant Staphylococcus aureus* (MRSA). This is a hybrid strain of the parent bacteria that is now becoming epidemic in our society. MRSA is so common now that a high percentage of the public harbors it. It is spread easily in hospitals, relationships, airplanes, etc. (Johnson, September 30, 2001). A few years ago, a patient of mine who worked in a high administrative position in a hospital told me that they cannot find surgical doctors and nurses who are not carriers. She also told me that they used to quarantine people in nursing homes who were carriers because of the threat to others. Now she says almost everyone is a carrier of this bacterium. I have seen much written on MRSA in the last few years because it is striking young people in their prime. Reports of this epidemic have been well known and documented in various medical reports as well as national media attention.

The second most common contributor is rhinovirus. Rhino is of Greek origin meaning nose. I find some people can harbor this virus for many years and, like any pathogen, it will cause an inflammatory pattern to exist.

Sinus enemy number three is *Moraxella catarrhalis*. It sounds like a cheese but it is a mycobacterium that will show up from time to time and cause, or contribute to, mucus production in the sinuses (Constantinescu, March 7, 2005).

Adenovirus and coronavirus are common winter viruses that cause colds. These can also get into the sinus cavities and play havoc. Antibiotics do nothing to kill viruses; in fact, they can sometimes drive a pathogen deeper into the system.

Most of the patients I have worked with that have been diagnosed with chronic sinusitis have been on the antibiotic therapy for years. They keep trying one after another without any permanent resolution. They all say it helped at first, but then it just kept coming back. Most bacteria like the *Staphylococcus* mentioned above will mutate in the presence of antibiotics. *Candida albicans* can also be a major contributor. *Candida albicans* is a yeast type fungus that becomes out of balance in our intestinal tract with the use of repeated courses of antibiotics. *Candida albicans* goes into the bloodstream from the intestinal tract and can enter the sinus cavities and stimulate inflammation. It also lowers our overall immune function so that other pathogens and allergies can take hold easier. Other fungi can also be causative agents such as various strains of *Aspergillus, Alternaria* and other strains of *Candida*. When antibiotics have failed to resolve the problem, then many ear, nose and throat specialists want to perform sinus surgery. They will actually go in and scrape the sinuses in order to clean them out. I have never personally met a patient who has had any long-term success with this procedure. Instead, many have repeated surgeries every few years with the same result. Surgery is these specialists only allopathic option if antibiotic therapy has failed.

Allergies

Allergies are the other cause of chronic sinusitis, though I see lingering pathogens as the primary cause. Sinusitis can be caused from allergens that people breathe. Environmental allergies such as dust, pollens, trees, grasses, mold, etc., can aggravate and inflame the sinuses and cause mucus to be produced. Many other allergens can produce sinus congestion, especially dairy foods and wheat. These two foods are mucus forming by themselves even if there is no allergy to them.

Also a diet high in sugar can aggravate *Candida albicans* and cause mucus production in the sinuses. This condition needs to be addressed by either eliminating the allergies that are causing it, or by going after the *Staphylococcus aureus* or other bugs in ways that do not include the use of antibiotics. These include allergy elimination techniques to address the allergies and protocols that enhance the immune/antigen responses to the lingering pathogens that are creating the inflammation.

Notes

Constantinescu, Michael, M.D. "Moraxella Catarrhalis Infections," eMedicine, Accessed March 7, 2005.
www.emedicine.com/med/topic1500.htm

Johnson, Linda A. "'Super Bugs' Infect the Super Healthy," *The (Tacoma, Washington) News Tribune*, September 30, 2001.

References

Murphy, Kate. "Bacteria's Expanding Reach Elicits Concern," *International Herald Tribune*, August 24, 2006.

Murray, Clinton, M.D. "Rhinoviruses," eMedicine, Accessed March 3, 2005.
www.emedicine.com/MED/topic2030.htm

Chapter 34: Ear and Eye Conditions

Ear and eye conditions can become chronic problems that can linger on and on without any relief. However, in some cases, they can turn into a major problem, as they have the potential for causing serious and permanent ear or eye damage. This is due to the delicate structures within the eyes and ears. The tympanic membrane in the ear, as well as the intricate structures of the eyes, such as the cornea and lens, can sustain irreversible damage if inflammation persists. The other factor is that the location of the eyes and ears lie in a vulnerable position for environmental and pathogenic invasion, as they are both exposed to the outside, with little protection.

Microbes and allergic substances can gain entry into the ears and eyes easily. The most common entry can come from airborne influences. The other factor has to do with the proximity of the sinuses to these areas. This close anatomical relationship sets up an interesting scenario in terms of transference of local migrating predators into both of these areas. The sinuses and the middle ear have a direct path, due to the eustachian tube, as it connects the sinuses to the middle ear drum. Any pathogen including bacteria, fungi or viruses all have a short stroll into the inner ear or eye. This is a perfect place to set up shop. The ear is like having a friendly cave in which migrating germs can find warmth and comfort. The eyes sit between the maxillary and frontal sinus cavities. Pathogenic entry into the eyes is in close proximity. This is like going over for dinner to your friends' house, right around the corner.

Ear and eye pathogens

Our familiar bacterial friend *Staphylococcus aureus* again heads the list. The sinuses are its favorite hangout, but it will invade the eyes and ears, whenever it pleases. Not all eye and ear problems all involve *Staphylococcus aureus*. However, if I were a gambling man, I would bet on it at least five out of ten times, and I would probably come out ahead.

The second most common pathogen in this area is a mycobacterium called *Moraxella catarrhalis*. This is a very small organism that seems to love invading the sinus cavities, eyes and ears. Other mycobacteria that have a tendency to invade the lungs can also be involved. *Streptococcus pneumoniae* is a very popular predator in the ears. Several other microbes can come to the party as well. These include the bacteria *Staphylococcus pyogenes*, *Pseudomonas aeruginosa* and *Haemophilus influenzae*. Another bug that occasionally shows up is *Mycoplasma fermentans*, which is now famous for its role in infectious arthritis. Somehow it also has a hankering for the eyes. Parasites also can invade both the eyes and ears. This can occur while swimming in natural lakes.

Fungi once in the sinuses can migrate to the eyes and ears causing low-grade inflammation.

Ear infections

Children seem to be the most vulnerable for getting ear infections. This is due to the structure of the eustachian tube during the early years. Because of its inverted position, the tube has a hard time draining. It becomes a perfect receptacle for collecting and breeding germs, especially bacteria. How many kids get early bacterial infections in their ears, and go to their pediatrician? In the past, most pediatricians were more than willing to get them started on antibiotics. The only problem is that once a child begins taking them, the child may come back often with more ear infections. This was discussed in Chapter 5 on The Disease Process. The antibiotics start knocking down the bacteria. However, because of the strong trend for bacteria to mutate into a cell wall deficient form, the variant strain survives, and now we have a stronger more resilient strain that will surely resurface its ugly little head sometime in the near future.

The other thing that will occur after a few rounds of antibiotic use is the start of *Candida albicans*, which immediately starts lowering immune function, thereby helping to support the reappearance of these little monsters.

After two or three rounds of antibiotics, the innocent child and unsuspecting parents have started that downward slide. This way of treating ear infections is quickly changing, as some pediatricians are finally starting to recognize that short-term relief with antibiotics usually leads to long-term problems. The change is occurring primarily due to numerous studies reported in medical reviews in the last few years. The research showed that children were only marginally better by taking antibiotics, in terms of short-term relief, compared to the children who took nothing at all. The ear infection usually resolved itself on its own within forty-eight to seventy-two hours.

Ear infection research

Robert S. Baltimore, M.D., co-director of the Pediatric Infectious Disease Training Program at the Yale University School of Medicine, spoke at an Infectious Diseases in Children Symposium in New York in October of 2006. Dr. Baltimore stated that an analysis of many studies on ear infections showed that 81 percent of them went away on their own without treatment, and that antibiotics raised the cure rate to only 94 percent. He also said that the liberal use of antibiotics came at a high price: It puts children at risk for future infections that would not respond to antibiotics. "Many of us believe that the use of broad spectrum antibiotics for ear infections has contributed to antibiotic resistance." Dr. Baltimore urged the attending pediatricians to not prescribe antibiotics in certain circumstances (Gilbert, November 27, 1996).

David A. Bergman, M.D., chairman of the Academy of Pediatricians Committee that establishes practice guidelines, stated, "For those kids whose symptoms aren't so bad, what's the point of antibiotics?" (Gilbert, November 27, 1996).

David Spiro, M.D., assistant professor of emergency medicine and pediatrics at Oregon Health and Science University, was involved in a yearlong study on ear infections and antibiotic use. The study concluded that there was no significant difference between the two groups of children, either taking antibiotics and those who refrained, with regard to fever, ear pain or return visits for medical care. Dr. Spiro said, "Antibiotic resistance is a global public health concern, and that over prescribing them for ear infections is part of that problem" (Oregon Health and Science University, September 12, 2005).

David McCormick, M.D., researcher and professor of pediatrics at the University of Texas, said, "Learning what is going on inside your child's ear is important for understanding why skipping the antibiotics may keep your child healthier."

What has happened as a result of this research is that pediatricians are now urged to advise parents to take a wait-and-see approach before prescribing antibiotics. Another interesting key factor is the discovery of biofilms, which are antibiotic resistant colonies of bacteria, that attach to surface tissue. They create a slime-like barrier that acts like a formidable defense mechanism, protecting the bacteria from eradication. A very high percentage of children treated with antibiotics for ear infections showed that colonies of these biofilms had developed inside their ear in response to the antibiotics used. In addition to this, new studies show that children treated with as little as one round of antibiotics in the first year for ear infections double their risk for getting asthma, as well as allergies. This is an interesting shift in thinking for traditional medicine. I applaud traditional medicine for this information finally coming to the forefront. I have been telling patients for more than ten years what these studies finally proved. However, I am not a medical doctor, so many times my thinking was not coming from "sound medical research" or not mentioned in any medical journal. Therefore, the patient followed the perceived medical wisdom, which included the liberal use of antibiotics.

Adult ear infections

Adults can also get ear infections. However, they usually occur with different symptoms. Vertigo is a common problem among older people. So is ringing of the ear or Meniere's disease. This so-called disease is explained in the Merck manual as a poorly understood disorder with an unknown cause, characterized by hearing loss, tinnitus (ringing in ears) and a feeling of fullness or pressure in the ear. It can cause long-term hearing loss if it persists. Nausea and vomiting can also occur during attacks.

If we break down the symptoms of this mysterious disease, we can see a pattern that logically evolves. We can then bring some common sense to what the cause of this disorder could actually be. Here are a few clues to help break this mystery wide open. We have a feeling of fullness and pressure in the ear. Could that be excess fluid being produced within the ear? What causes excess fluid to be produced in a cavity of any kind? If you had excess fluid in your knee joint, would the signs possibly be swelling and pressure? What is the definition of inflammation? Pressure, swelling, redness and pain. When inflammation is long term, what happens to the structure that the inflammation is residing in? Does it deteriorate? Could damage to the delicate structures of the eardrum from the long-term inflammation cause progressive hearing loss? Since the middle ear has neurological and sensory connections to balance, could there possibly be a connection to the vertigo? The stomach meridian runs just anterior to the ear. Stomach 6 (an acupuncture point) sits just in front of the opening of the eardrum. Stomach symptoms such as nausea and vomiting may be a reflection of this connection. This is the last and final clue; the ringing is the poor middle ear alarm going off, screaming, "Hey guys, someone wake up, I have a _____ in my ear! Can anyone please get it out?" The fill-in answer is, of course, a bug or microbe. Have we just unraveled the mysterious, unknown, perplexing problem that for years has baffled the great medical minds?

Some people also report chronic itching in the ears, as well as a feeling like there is something crawling around in the ear. Can we make a guess about what it could probably be? Some also report a feeling of fluid inside the ear. The same bugs that cause children's ear problems also can cause adults' problems in most cases. The reason adults have fewer earaches is due to the development of the eustachian tube. Adults are more prone to other symptoms from the inflammation, instead of the pain that accompanies ear infections.

Other ear pathogens

Adeno, corona, respiratory syncytial and rhino viruses all have the ability to enter the ear. They are common winter cold viruses that congregate in the head area and sinuses, thereby making their way into the ear. These viruses are less common causes of ear infection, but they cannot be ruled out. Swimming in lakes can be a hazard because various amoebas and other types of parasites, as well as various bacteria, can enter an open ear canal and treat it like they just bought their first new home. Yes, they unfortunately can become homebodies in your house.

Eye infections

Eye infections are quite common, and can come from a wide range of pathogens. However, various bacteria, much like in the ears, are the common culprits. Heading up the bacteria list are *Staphylococcus aureus*, *Pseudomonas aeruginosa*, and the newcomer *Chlamydia trachomatis*. The mycobacterium *Moraxella catarrhalis* also is involved. Adenovirus, cytomegalovirus and herpes simplex 1 and 2 can infect the eyes as well. However, there are a few other potential candidates that seem to like the eyes. Fungal infections seem to be common, especially with contact lenses. Numerous types of fungi, including various strains of *Candida*, can invade the eyes.

One of my early rheumatoid arthritis patients also had a concurrent eye problem. It seemed her left eye had been deteriorating for over a year, as she had lost about 50 percent of her vision in that eye. She said that her rheumatologist had told her that some people with rheumatoid arthritis also have concurrent vision deterioration. The doctor said that she could possibly lose her eyesight within the next few years if it continued to deteriorate at the present rate. I believe the same bug that is causing rheumatoid arthritis, which is *Mycoplasma fermentans*, can also cause an eye infection, with subsequent deterioration. After working with her awhile, both her arthritis and eye problems cleared up simultaneously.

Another interesting event happened a few years ago. A patient of mine came in complaining that her eyesight had drastically deteriorated within a short time. I had worked with her in the past on some other issues. However, it had been awhile since she had been in. She had gone to a local optometrist, who had done extensive testing, and had taken some elaborate retinal eye photos. The optometrist had no clue as to why the deterioration was happening. He told her that if it continued, she could lose the sight in her eye. He had no plan of action, so she was a bit alarmed and stressed because of it. She was a nurse who made home visits on a regular basis.

I thought she may have picked up some type of lingering pathogen that could be residing in her eye causing the deterioration. My Chinese medicine diagnosis was heat in the affected eye causing pain. I supported her immune system and eye with acupuncture so it could better respond to any pathogen that was affecting her eye. Within a few sessions her eyesight began to improve. After three sessions, she reported that her eyesight was almost back to normal. She then went back to her optometrist following the third session and reported what had transpired. He took some new photos and was shocked and surprised by what had happened. The before and after photos revealed a huge shift in how the eye looked. The pictures revealed that the eye was returning to its former healthy self. After a few more sessions the eyesight returned to normal. The optometrist somehow could not make the connection that possibly a common bacterium such as *Staph aureus* or another pathogen could cause the sudden deterioration of her eyesight. He was also surprised that acupuncture could make such quick changes. To be totally honest, I was amazed that he was so surprised. It was an amazing experience for the nurse and me, and a great educational gift for all involved.

Neurological eye problems

The next two experiences I had with eye disorders involved neurological eye problems. I mentioned these in Chapter 28 on Neurological Disorders. The symptoms were of the twitching variety. When you see twitching in any area of the body, you always figure that it could be a neurologically based problem. The first incident involved a person who was a public speaker. He had a major twitching problem that had been there for ten years. I supported his immune system and eye with acupuncture. After three sessions, he did not notice any difference, and felt this type of treatment was a waste of time and money. I encouraged him to give it a bit more time. Each treatment that followed seemed to decrease the eye twitch. After six treatments, he said his twitching had decreased more than 75 percent. I recently saw him, and his eye was still was doing well; it had been two years since our sessions.

A much younger gentlemen came to me with the same issue about six months later. He had been to several conventional doctors, including a neurologist. They had no answer for the twitch, except to medicate him, which he refused. I also supported his immune system in a similar way as above. After six treatments, his eyes stopped twitching. He said, "Thank you, sir," and I have not heard from him since.

The role of pathogens

Recently, one of my favorite elderly patients came to me with dark circles that suddenly appeared under her eyes. She also complained that her eyes also felt heavy. Dark circles under the eyes are usually due to allergic reactions. However, pathogenic invasion, especially in the eye area, can bring them on as well. She was an extremely healthy eighty-four year old, going on thirty something, and did not seem to have many sensitivities. I diagnosed her as having heat in the head and eye area. Because it came on suddenly, I thought that a lingering pathogen may have been the culprit. I supported her immune system and eye with acupuncture. After only a few sessions, both of her eye symptoms cleared up. The dark circles left, as well as the heaviness.

Red, dry or watery eyes

I have worked with several people who have red or dry eyes. This is a reflection of too much heat in the interior of the body. Usually chronic pathogenic infection is the underlying cause, because the heat is a byproduct of the inflammation process.

An elegant older women came to me a few years ago with chronic constipation, occasional intestinal pain and chronic dry eyes. She had been a long-time patient of traditional medicine. She was on a stool softener for her constipation, as well as having to constantly use eye drops to keep her eyes lubricated. Her husband was a retired pharmaceutical salesman. They were both health conscious, and had exhausted all traditional medicine had to offer. During the initial interview, I made a remark purposely, just to see her reaction; that the constipation and dry eyes were probably from the same source. She gave me a funny look, like, "Yeah right, show me to the exit door." Most traditional as well as many nontraditional medical experts would probably have agreed with her as well. Before she got up to leave, I went on to explain to her that constipation is almost always a reflection of food sensitivities or one or more lingering pathogens in the intestines, which is creating heat, thereby drying up the stools. She got that part pretty quick, but then responded by saying, "Well, what does that have to do with my eyes?" I laughed a bit, as I was trying to have some fun with her, but went on to reply, "If you follow your intestinal tract back up from your chronically inflamed gut, where does it end up?" I was really enjoying the suspense, to see if, and when, she could figure it out with enough of the right clues.

The mouth was finally discovered to be the correct anatomical upper exit hole. I went on to explain, "This heat, coming from the intestines will rise upward and make its way into the head area." Heat has a tendency to naturally rise. This is also basic

Chinese medicine theory. Heat from the liver and/or intestines can rise and create heat in the head. The eyes are the headlights of the head. Any chronic increase of heat in the head will usually show up as redness or dryness in the eyes. Heat traveling upward without a lower exit point has to go somewhere. Because most of us hopefully keep our mouths closed most of the time, much of this heat is simply transferred to the head. My patient pondered that for a few moments and said, "You know, that actually makes sense." We went on to get rid of both the intestinal heat and dry eyes simultaneously.

Watery eyes can be pathogenic as well. However, I tend to see environmental allergies, such as pollen, grasses, dust, etc., as the main culprits behind this issue.

The most interesting eye case happened within the last year. This darling little eight-year-old girl came to me with some intestinal problems and occasional blurriness in the eyes, which seemed to be progressively getting worse. Her mom had taken her to an eye specialist, who had few answers for what was going on. She referred her to a top pediatric ophthalmologist for extensive testing. I started working with her on both problems. Her parents had been prior patients of mine, and had some life changing experiences. We had a working trust level, which makes my job easier. It amazes me that most people will exhaust every possible avenue with the traditional medical system, but have such a short fuse with alternative methods. Thank God for those who have the courage to be self-thinkers.

After a visit or two, the eight-year-old's mom came to me in a panic. She was expressing major concern about her daughter's eyes, as the deterioration was rapidly progressing. The symptoms had suddenly worsened within just a couple of days, to the point of her losing total eyesight for brief periods of time. Her mom had called the Children's Hospital in Seattle to get an emergency appointment. Things had turned very serious and scary in a short period of time. After I did some extensive Chinese medicine testing with her, I supported her immune system and eye with acupuncture. I suspected that possibly a lingering pathogen may be affecting the optic nerve. Following the first session, her eyesight started to improve. She returned to the prior sporadic episodes of blurred vision, instead of the temporary blindness. Following the second session, her blurred vision episodes were becoming less frequent. After four sessions, the blurriness halted, and her eyesight returned to normal. Her family and I were both elated. I took a big breath and sigh of relief.

Understanding the role that a lingering pathogen, such as a simple bacterium or mycobacterium, can play in causing deterioration of the dopamine receptors in the base of the brain in Parkinson's disease, as well as their role in eye and ear infections, is essential. The proximity of these breeding areas makes it an easy transition in causing various eye infectious disorders, including blindness. Remember that most infections in the body that cause serious illness are of the low-grade chronic variety. We have been conditioned by the medical experts to think of infection as being associated with mostly acute illness. This is simply not true. Rapid or progressive deterioration of eyesight can be either acute or chronic.

How many people in this country live with a chronic sinus infection? The delicate structures of the eyes will deteriorate much more quickly than most other body parts, including the sinus cavities, if infection goes untreated. That is why people get mucus production with sinus infections. This response is used to protect against damage to the sinuses. The eyes do not have as good a mechanism built in for protection.

Chronic eye infections are often misdiagnosed. Doctors of all types can get hung up in the name the symptom game, and trying to figure out which category those symptoms fit into. Then we have a label for it, and everyone is happy, right? This is why compartment medicine in any medical or health related field has so much limitation. Category placement usually has little to do with the cause and effect, and ignores the obvious question of what is really going on underneath the symptoms. I may be different from most. I would rather have a doctor who understands what is underlying my symptoms and how to get rid of the actual cause of them, instead of being tagged with a fancy name for my symptoms without any understanding of what caused them in the first place. This is why I never was a good patient with traditional-thinking health professionals. I often asked all the "wrong" questions that the doctor could not answer, such as, "What is causing this and how do we get rid of it?"

Eye problems and Chinese medicine

Eye problems are associated with liver dysfunction in Chinese medicine. This is true in some cases that are not related to direct eye infection. Red or dry eyes are an indicator of too much heat in the liver or intestines, which will also show up as dryness or redness in the eyes or tongue. That is why the tongue is looked at as part of the Traditional Chinese Medical model of diagnosis. Whenever a person says, "I am always thirsty," this is a major clue that there is too much heat trapped within the interior of the body. As that heat rises, it will show up as heat somewhere in the head. Dry eyes are also a reflection of a general yin deficiency of some type, usually liver yin. This means the cooling mechanisms of the body are not circulating the fluids properly, allowing too much heat in the interior. This comes from a deficiency creating the heat, instead of an excess. It is much like a plugged radiator that cannot cool the engine. Again, the heat shows up in the head, such as the eyes or tongue, which are a reflection of the dryness within the system.

Using acupuncture points and herbs to clear out the internal heat and support the yin organs such as the spleen, kidneys and liver, thereby helping the body to cool down, is always a positive direction in which to go. Supporting the immune system in its ability to remove the lingering pathogens, either within the interior or localized in the head area, is often the key to treating the root cause, thereby achieving lasting results. This is why I believe that acupuncture and immune support together can be a great recipe for success in some of these difficult cases.

Natural remedies

There are also natural remedies that can be used to decrease infection. Garlic and oregano oils have been used with some success. However, you may end up smelling like an Italian meal. Several companies manufacture natural ear remedies that target the bacteria and inflammation. I would recommend this approach, especially at the onset of any ear infection.

The future

Antibiotic therapies will always have their place in the treatment of certain disorders. However, I believe the shift in thinking by the traditional medical thinkers is only the beginning of what we will ultimately understand in the future.

Sinus infections need to be the next area of scientific investigation that will prove similar ineffective results when using antibiotic therapies as the studies have proven with ear infections. Namely, that bacteria create biofilms and mutation in order to defend themselves and survive in response to antibiotics. These critters have figured out the game. The game is being played on many fields within your body. What is the difference if the playing field is your ears, eyes, sinuses or anywhere else? In the future, I hope that more patients will consider other options, before they think about taking antibiotics.

Notes

Gilbert, Susan. "New Questions on Antibiotics for Ear Infections," *The New York Times*, November 27, 1996.

"Taking a 'Wait-and-See' Approach to Childhood Ear Infections Is as Effective as Immediate Antibiotics," Oregon Health and Science University, September 12, 2005. www.ohsu.edu/ohsuedu/newspub/releases/09120ear.cfm

"Wait and Hear: Letting Ear Infections Clear Without Antibiotics," Iconocast, June 6, 2005.
www.iconocast.com/News_Files/HNewsxx_xx_m3News5.htm

References

"Adenovirus Serotypes 8, 19, and 37," Stanford University, Accessed June 23, 2007.
www.stanford.edu/group/virus/adeno/2000/eyeinfections.html

"Chronic Middle Ear Infections Linked to Resistant Biofilm," Medical College of Wisconsin, July 11, 2006.
www.mcw.edu/display/router.asp?docid=17667

Constantinescu, Michael, M.D. "Moraxella Catarrhalis Infections," eMedicine, Accessed March 14, 2005.
www.emedicine.com/MED/topic1500.htm

Deadman, Peter and Mazin Al-Khafaji. *A Manual of Acupuncture.* Vista, California: Eastland Press, 1998.

"Eye Infections," Wilmer Eye Institute, Accessed June 23, 2007.
www.hopkinsmedical.org/wilmer/Conditions/index.html

Fratkin, Jake Paul, OMD, L.Ac. "Pediatric Ear Infections," *News From Golden Flower,* Fall 2004.

Griva, Ven. "Pediatricians Adopt New Strategy for Fighting Ear Infections," *The Homesteader,* Northern Colorado Edition, April 2006.

"Herpes Simplex Eye Infections," Steen Hall Eye Institute, Accessed June 23, 2007.
www.steen-hall.com/hsimplex.html

"Increase in Drug Resistance for Common Bacterium Termed 'Rocket Ship' Based on National Study," Science Daily, October 4, 1997.
www.sciencedaily.com/releases/1997/10/971004092328.html

Kinonen, Judie. "Study: Non-drug Approach Works for Most Ear Infections," The

University of Texas Medical Branch, June 7, 2005.
www.utmb.edu/impact/stories/2005/05JUNE6/watchandwait.htm

"More Fungal Eye Infections," Johns Hopkins Bayview Medical Center, June 14, 2006.
www.hopkinsbayview.org/healthcarenews06/060614eye.html

Murphy, Kate. "Bacteria's Expanding Reach Elicits Concern," *International Herald Tribune*, August 24, 2006.

Noble, Elizabeth, N.D. "How to Stop the Agony of an Ear Infection Within Minutes," Wholistic Therapy Centre, Accessed June 23, 2007.
www.wholistictherapycentre.com/ear-ache/ear-infection.htm.

Paulson, Tom. "Antibiotics Prompt Bacteria 'Walls,'" *The Olympian,* August 25, 2005.

Stevens, Corey. "Ear Infection Complications on the Rise," ScienceDaily, September 15, 1998.
www.sciencedaily.com/releases/1998/09/980914145029.htm

"'Watch and Wait'–A Shift in Approach to Kids' Ear Infections," Pediatrics/Children's Health News, June 6, 2005.

Chapter 35: Chronic Fatigue Syndrome

Chronic fatigue syndrome is not really a syndrome, rather it is nothing more than an effect. This term has been used the last ten years or so implying that it is a mysterious type of disease. Many people who have been diagnosed with this syndrome have no idea how they got it. It just seemed to show up one day or came on slowly. Traditional medical experts have no answer for this syndrome, except to recommend long-term rest.

Acupuncture is helpful, along with certain key supplements and herbs. The person may be helped to some degree by these means, but the underlying fatigue is still there in many cases. The reason supplements are not the total answer is because the syndrome was not caused by not taking the supplements. Natural medicine is a better approach, but there is a huge piece missing from this puzzle.

A perplexing problem

The only known cause of this syndrome, according to the medical experts, is Epstein-Barr virus. They are correct that this virus can cause chronic fatigue. However, many people have chronic fatigue without this virus in their system. I have found that chronic fatigue is usually an accumulation of pathogens, nutritional deficiencies and sensitivities, along with organ and glandular dysfunction, including the thyroid and adrenal glands. Chinese medicine looks at the kidneys as the source of energy and endurance in the body. This is true, due to the kidney's relationship with the adrenal glands. Many natural medicine practitioners focus on the adrenal and thyroid glands as a way to support the chronically fatigued individual. Low-functioning adrenal and thyroid glands can contribute to fatigue. This can be helpful, but I find it is usually only a piece of the puzzle, as there are bigger fires burning. Nutritional deficiencies such as iron, B complex and certain amino acids can also play a role. How do we know what the true cause is, if there are so many pieces to the puzzle?

The role of pathogens

I believe that multiple lingering pathogens are the primary cause in chronic fatigue. The amount of fatigue produced by a certain pathogen depends on many factors.

The type of pathogen is the first key. For instance, a lingering mycoplasma or spirochete such as in Lyme disease can cause a lot more fatigue than a simple bacterium in most cases. A mycoplasma can greatly decrease the functioning of the mitochondria by stealing lipids that cause the mitochondria to lose electrons. It is like a battery that is losing its juice very quickly without being able to replenish itself on a cellular level. This is one of the key factors in fatiguing syndromes. Most people with mycoplasma infection are exhausted at a cellular level. A bacterium in the middle ear may cause an earache, but not have much of an effect on the overall energetic picture, because it is being contained there. However, the same bacterium in the lungs can have a larger effect on energy levels, as the lungs are a key organ involved in the exchange of oxygen. Weak lungs lead to decreased oxygen uptake and subsequent fatigue.

Secondly, the quantity of the pathogen plays a huge factor. A pathogen that is contained in a certain area will have less effect than one whose numbers have grown and have migrated to several areas of the body, including the blood, lymph and organs. This is when systemic weakening and fatigue set in.

The third factor is how many different pathogens are present within the system, called the multiple pathogenic factor. This is when the body really starts to become beaten down. Not only can a patient get chronic fatigue, but chronic disease can set in as well. This sets up the environment for the potential to contract cancer, autoimmune conditions, cardiovascular disease, diabetes and a host of other chronic conditions. The amount in numbers, varieties of pathogens and locations are the primary factors in fatiguing illnesses.

The fourth factor involves the liver, spleen, kidneys and adrenal glands. Pathogens cause a long-term weakening of these organs because of the toxic byproducts that are released as a result of the constant presence of pathogens and the immune system's attacks upon them. The liver and kidneys play key roles in the detoxification process of these toxic chemicals and free radicals. The adrenals and kidneys are weakened by the constant internal stress that goes on nonstop within the body. Any key organ that is a host for a pathogenic invasion will be greatly weakened. Multiple organ invasions lead to overall systemic exhaustion. According to Chinese medicine, when the kidneys are depleted, the body's energy and sexual desire are lowered. See Chapter 8: Organ Degradation.

Nutritional deficiencies

I mentioned B complex and iron as key nutritional components for feeling energetic. Many people take an excess of these nutrients thinking this is the answer, but they can still show a deficiency when tested. The reason is that they are sensitive to, or allergic to, these substances, so their body has difficulty metabolizing them. Sensitivity to B_6, B_{12} and folic acid can cause a blood deficiency pattern. A similar problem with iron will cause anemia. Any combination of these factors will affect energy levels, as well as mood. Many people who have had these nutrients, such as iron and vitamin B complex, repatterned back into their systems will show sufficient levels for the first time in their lives. The body is now able to absorb these key nutrients and energy levels rise. Coenzyme Q10, lipoic acid and pyruvic acid are key support components of the Krebs cycle. This is your energy production cycle. Any sensitivity to these can cause a deficiency, which can impede your energy production as well. Multiple allergies can drain your energy, as the body constantly has to react to a stressful internal environment. I see the above nutrient deficiencies and allergies as being a definite contributor and a secondary cause of chronic fatigue in most cases.

A combination of problems

When you put any combination of pathogens, allergies, nutritional deficiencies and toxic overload together with organ and glandular degradation/dysfunction, the body will be in a fatigued state. The severity depends on many factors. The more pathogens, allergies and toxins a person has the more they will experience fatigue, as well as other symptoms. Genetics, stress, injuries and nutrition are some of the other factors that play a key role as well. The bottom line is that fatigue is nothing more than an effect of a larger picture.

The above scenarios are possibly some of the key pieces of the puzzle. Once they are brought into balance, the so-called syndrome vanishes and normal functioning and energy naturally return, as there is nothing impeding the body's function. In Chinese medicine, it is referred to as having good qi.

References

Deadman, Peter and Mazin Al-Khafaji. *A Manual of Acupuncture*. Vista, California: Eastland Press, 1998.

Guthrie, Michael, R.PH. "Mycoplasmas: The Missing Link in Fatiguing Illness," *Alternative Medicine*, September 2001.

Nicolson, Garth L., Ph.D. "Autoimmune Illnesses and Degenerative Diseases," The Institute for Molecular Medicine, Accessed June 26, 2005. www.immed.org/illness/fatigue_autoimmune_illness_research.html

Nicolson, Garth L., Ph.D. "Chronic Fatigue Illnesses," The Institute for Molecular Medicine," Accessed June 26, 2005.
www.immed.org/illness/infectious_disease_research.html

Nicolson, Garth L., Ph.D. "Chronic Infectious Diseases," The Institute for Molecular Medicine, Accessed June 26, 2005.
www.immed.org/illness/fatigue_illness_research.html

Nicolson, Garth L., Ph.D. "VA Confirms Nicholson's Data on Chronic Infections in Gulf War Illness Patients," The Institute for Molecular Medicine, March 25, 2000.
www.immed.org/illness/whatsnew/news00-3-25.html

Sinha, Gunjan. "Gulf War Illness: Psychological?" *Popular Science*, April 1999.

Chapter 36: Chronic Joint Pain

Chronic joint pain is such a common problem I thought it was important enough to have its own chapter. Years ago while practicing as a massage therapist, I was always puzzled when I would work on someone who had chronic joint pain and be able to get only temporary relief. It was always very frustrating. I specialized in auto accidents and chronic pain. I had training in various modalities. I have also taught anatomy, physiology, structural and functional kinesiology, and injury rehabilitation from a soft tissue approach. I thought I had a handle on any possible cause of soft tissue dysfunction. Many chiropractors, physical therapists and massage therapists may feel just as frustrated as I did. I was puzzled when the joint I was working on would get somewhat better, but the pain would soon return or a new joint would flare up for no apparent reason. I am aware that previous injuries with joint damage can cause this. However, these people had no previous injury; or at least if they did have a prior injury, it was out of proportion to the symptoms they were feeling.

Spinal problems are also part of joint dysfunction. When a chiropractor adjusts a patient to the point of knowing that the spine is in balance and does not see any deformities or damage to the spine, but the pain still persists, then something else has to be causing the joint dysfunction. The spine may, for some reason, go out of balance and need an adjustment on a regular basis without any logical reason for it. The adjustment may help temporarily, but again the patient soon returns because the pain is back again. The chiropractor verifies the misalignment and adjusts again and again. This can go on for years without either the patient or the chiropractor understanding the underlying cause of the subluxation. The chiropractor is doing exactly what he and other chiropractors were taught in school.

The role of pathogens

The underlying cause of not only the chronic pain, but the misalignment as well, may be the presence of an underlying pathogen causing a low-grade inflammatory condition to persist. This low-grade inflammation causes the muscles to tighten and the nerves to fire, which pulls on the adjoining vertebrae causing subluxation. When it is adjusted, this takes some pressure off the joint and the patient may get some temporary relief. However, because of the underlying problem, the joint soon reverts back to the previous state and the process continues. I have witnessed my patients' need for adjustments dramatically decrease or completely cease once the underlying cause of the inflammation is addressed. It was inflammation of the joints and spine caused by a lingering pathogen that was the underlying cause of the pain and a regular need for adjustments.

I often see patients that believe their pain is caused from a previous injury. With further questioning I find that the apparent injury, which supposedly caused this, was a very minor one and does not seem to justify the amount and frequency of pain associated with that injury. My experience indicates that pathogens tend to migrate to injured tissue. Intracellular pathogens are carried by the immune system to the injury site and become a lingering pathogen once the initial crisis is over. The presence of pathogens can prevent the damaged tissue from healing and may cause the inflammation to persist long after the injury.

Another factor to be aware of is related to joint damage that shows up on an X-ray where there has been a previous injury. There is a chance that the actual injury was not responsible for that amount of damage. The health professional diagnosing the condition can ascertain the damage from an X-ray or magnetic resonance imaging (MRI), and assume that the pain is a direct reflection of what is visible, caused by the initial injury. However, a person may have a lingering pathogen that was causing the chronic inflammation, which in turn damaged the tissue. The pain may be caused from two sources: one is from the apparent trauma to the joint, and the other is from the ongoing inflammation that the lingering pathogen creates, which adds to the damage. That is why the verification of the damaged joint does not necessarily justify the chronic pain, due to the unseen pathogenic presence. Joint pain can be a complex issue, especially when it becomes chronic. There are many factors to consider.

Many different pathogens have been implicated in degenerative joint diseases. The most common are: *Mycoplasma fermentans* and the bacteria *Propioni acnes* and *Yersinia*. These three bugs are responsible for the majority of non-injury related chronic joint dysfunction. (See Chapter 21: Mycoplasmas for more details.) *Propioni acnes* is not as well known. *Alternative Medicine Digest* offered an excellent article on this bacterium in issue No. 18, entitled "Rheumatoid Arthritis and Multiple Sclerosis, the Cause May Be in the Blood" by Philip Hoekstra, Ph.D., which sheds much needed light on the fact that these living organisms can be physically seen in the blood. He found that in virtually all the cases of rheumatoid arthritis, the patient had significant amounts of *Propioni acnes* in their altered cell wall deficient state. (See Chapter 19: Cell Wall Deficient Pathogens for further information on this phenomenon). G.A. Denys at Wayne State University in Detroit, Michigan, first identified this bacterium in 1981. Hoekstra explains how this bacterium is passed transplacentally from mother to fetus, and how this may be responsible for rheumatoid arthritis (Hoekstra, 1996). Lida Mattman, Ph.D., also of Wayne State University, extracted the bacterium from the synovial fluid of human arthritis patients and injected it into chicken embryos. The chickens then exhibited symptoms of arthritis. Various bacteria that have also been identified in joint pathology include *Listeria, Micrococcus rheumaticus, Streptococcus* and *Staphylococcus*. Other common intestinal bacteria also can be implicated. These include *Yersinia, Chlamydia, Shigella, Campylobacter and Salmonella. Yersinia*, in particular, seems to be the most common of these intestinal bacteria. The occurrence of this is due to these bacteria entering the intestinal tract and making their way into the bloodstream through the gut lining. The increased prevalence of this happening is in relationship to the amount of damage that the intestinal mucosa has previously sustained. This damage is due to the overuse of antibiotics as well as the invasion of other microbes, especially parasites that have previously damaged this valuable gut barrier. (See Chapter 15: Leaky Gut Syndrome.) This is another reason why the use of antibiotics has increased the instances of arthritic conditions. The proper term for this is reactive or infective arthritis. Any single bacterium or mycobacterium, in addition those mentioned above, can also be involved in causing chronic joint pain (Mattman, 2001).

Other potential invaders can be fungi such as *Candida albicans*, mycobacteria, parasites, *Borrelia burgdorferi* (a spirochete that causes Lyme disease) and nanobacteria. These pathogens need to be considered also, as they can invade the joints. Viruses tend to be the least likely habitant. The reason certain pathogens seem to invade joints more freely than others has to do with their structure. *Mycoplasma fermentans* has some of our own joint structure incorporated into its membrane surface. This gives it the ability to bind much more easily into joint tissue and also use the advantage of mimicry, which is the ability to mimic this structure. The immune system then becomes confused, due to seeing its own tissue as a potential area of attack. When these attacks take place, the pathogens are rooted so deeply into the body's joint tissue that the immune system cannot quite extract them out, but keeps trying, because that is its job. *Mycoplasma salivarius* also may be a culprit in chronic joint etiology.

Heavy metals and allergies

Heavy metals such as mercury, lead and cadmium should not be overlooked. They can leak into joints and cause the immune system to attack it much like a pathogen.

Allergies also can cause joint pain, as well as muscle pain. Wheat, eggs and dairy foods are common reactants that can play a major role in joint pain. In Chinese medicine, the meridians pass through all the joints of our body. Any meridian can be blocked by an allergen and the body's subsequent reaction to it can cause any joint along its path to become blocked or weakened.

The future

People may have been diagnosed with arthritis, bursitis or tendonitis. These all refer to where the inflammation is present. It is a category of a symptom and its effect. Instead, all that really matters is, "What is the cause and how can we get rid of it?" Symptomatic treatment protocols for pathogenic-induced joint problems will only give the patient temporary relief at best. Pathogenic joint invasion in allopathic medicine is referred to as septic or infective arthritis. Any nurse, doctor or surgeon who works in a hospital knows that various pathogens, especially *Staph* and *Strep* in a hospital environment can take over joints, organs, the brain or the entire body, for that matter, even causing death in some cases as the antibiotic therapy is rendered ineffective.

I believe that most arthritis is actually infective arthritis. More and more research and books are uncovering this truth. Why the medical profession is not welcoming this information has to do with rigidity, lack of understanding and most of all, that game called "disease management." Why should a cure be found if symptoms can continue to be treated? This makes sense from a financial point of view. The only ones who lose are the patients who suffer needlessly.

During my final editing stages of this book, I discovered a wonderful book called *Rheumatoid Arthritis: The Infection Connection* by Katherine M. Poehlmann, Ph.D. This book has great information on infective arthritis and the reasons why change is so difficult within the medical profession. She does acknowledge the financial aspects of the disease as being a key component of concern. David Brownstein, M.D., has also written a book on this subject identifying chronic infection as a primary cause of arthritis. I hope that more information like these books and others that have been previously written on this subject will someday give medical and alternative doctors the awareness to make this information available to the general public. In this way, we could see this disease process and suffering patients in a much different light.

Notes

Hoekstra, Philip, Ph.D. "Rheumatoid Arthritis and Multiple Sclerosis—The Cause May Be in the Blood," *Alternative Medicine Digest*, Issue No. 18, 1996.

Mattman, Lida H. *Cell Wall Deficient Forms–Stealth Pathogens*. Boca Raton, Florida: CRC Press LLC, 2001.

References

Abramson, John, M.D. *Overdosed America: The Broken Promise of American Medicine*. New York: Harper Perennial, 2005.

Brownstein, David, M.D. *Overcoming Arthritis*. West Bloomfield, Michigan: Medical Alternatives Press, 2001.

Centers for Disease Control and Prevention. "Shigellosis," Accessed June 5, 2004. www.cdc.gov/ncidod/dbmd/diseaseinfo/shigellosis_g.htm

Guthrie, Michael, R.PH. "Mycoplasmas: The Missing Link in Fatiguing Illness," *Alternative Medicine*, September 2001.

Moynihan, Ray and Alan Cassels. *Selling Sickness: How the World's Biggest Pharmaceutical Companies Are Turning Us All Into Patients*. New York: Nation Books, 2005.

Nicolson, Garth L., Ph.D. "Autoimmune Illnesses and Degenerative Diseases," The Institute for Molecular Medicine, Accessed June 26, 2005. www.immed.org/illness/fatigue_autoimmune_illness_research.html

Nicolson, Garth L., Ph.D. "Chronic Fatigue Illnesses," The Institute for Molecular Medicine, Accessed June 26, 2005. www.immed.org/illness/infectious_disease_research.html

Nicolson, Garth L., Ph.D. "Chronic Infectious Diseases," The Institute for Molecular Medicine, Accessed June 26, 2005. www.immed.org/illness/fatigue_illness_research.html

Nicolson, Garth L., Ph.D. "VA Confirms Nicholson's Data on Chronic Infections in Gulf War Illness Patients," The Institute for Molecular Medicine, March 25, 2000. www.immed.org/illness/whatsnew/news00-3-25.html

Poehlmann, Katherine M., Ph.D. *Rheumatoid Arthritis: The Infection Connection–Targeting and Treating the Cause of Chronic Illness*. Rolling Hills Estates, California: Satori Press, 2002.

"Reactive Arthritis," The Arthritis Society, Accessed April 1, 2007. www.arthritis.ca/types%20of%20arthritis/reactive%20arthritis/default.asp?s=1

"Reactive Arthritis," eMedicine, Accessed April 1, 2007. www.emedicine.com/emerg/byname/reactive-arthritis.htm

"The Road Back," A Review of the Book by Thomas MacPherson Brown, M.D., and Henry Scammell. *Nutrition News*, Vol. XVII, No. 7, 1993.

Scammell, Henry. *The New Arthritis Breakthrough: The Only Medical Therapy Clinically Proven to Produce Long-Term Improvement and Remission*, New York: M. Evans and Company Inc., 1998.

Sinha, Gunjan. "Gulf War Illness: Psychological?" *Popular Science*, April 1999.

Stanley, Doris. "Arthritis From Foodborne Bacteria?" *Agricultural Research*, October 1996.

Svenungsson, B. "Editorial: Reactive Arthritis," *British Medical Journal*, March 12, 1994.

Chapter 37: Chronic Muscle Pain/Fibromyalgia

Fibromyalgia means muscle pain and inflammation. Many theories on the causes are related to muscle metabolism, the Krebs cycle and magnesium. The Krebs cycle is the blueprint for how energy is processed within a muscle cell. Krebs cycle dysfunction causes muscle pain and fatigue. Books and articles have been written and a host of supplements designed to increase the components of what is supposedly missing. Key components of the Krebs cycle are coenzyme Q10, lipoic acid, pyruvic acid and malic acid, which are produced in pill form and available in most health food stores. The theory is to give your body something that it is supposedly missing. Magnesium is also added to the protocol, because it will relax muscles.

The physiological definition of the function of the Krebs cycle is how energy is produced within your body, but more specifically within your muscles. There are a half dozen or so components of this process that end up producing adenosine triphosphate (ATP). Any lack of key components such as the ones mentioned above can cause muscle pain, fatigue and energy deficiency problems. This sounds good on paper, but in my opinion any benefits from this postulation have been marginal at best.

The role of pathogens

Fibromyalgia is usually not a deficiency problem. In most cases, it is caused by a lingering pathogen. There are exceptions that will be discussed. When pathogens reside in the muscles, they create inflammation, which clogs the system and interferes with muscle metabolism. They block, or greatly hinder, the Krebs cycle's ability to produce ATP by damaging or hindering the mitochondria of the cell. They cause an overburdening of cellular debris to occur. This will overload the lymphatic system's ability to drain the muscle, which in turn blocks the influx of fresh blood, and nutrients that the muscle cells need to produce energy. This all leads to an over acidic and depleted oxygen environment. This becomes a cascading effect that starts with pathogenic entry into the muscle tissue at the cellular level. The Krebs cycle's inability to function properly then becomes an effect of the whole scenario. Taking supplements to somehow replenish this depleted effect is the reason why most people usually have little positive change with this approach. They may feel marginal improvement at best, as long as they are taking the supplement protocol. This, for some, is better than doing nothing at all.

Chinese medicine

Chinese medicine theory associates a constrained or stagnant liver as a contributor to muscle pain and weakness. This makes little sense to the American medical model. However, I can attest that there is a definite correlation between a person who has liver stagnation and muscle problems. The liver controls the sinews and allows the blood to flow unhindered. Therefore, a healthy free flowing liver allows fresh circulating blood to move freely through muscles and joints, as it nourishes and aids in the removal of waste products. Certain acupuncture points, along with herbal remedies, can support this process and reduce the muscle fatigue and soreness.

Leaky gut syndrome

There is a belief by some that fibromyalgia can be attributed to leaky gut syndrome. (See Chapter 15: Leaky Gut Syndrome for more information.) The rationale behind this is that a leaky gut will allow pathogenic invasion or toxic ingestants and byproducts directly into the bloodstream from the damaged gut wall, along with particles such as undigested foods, especially protein. Once inside the bloodstream they are absorbed into a muscle cell and begin the inflammation process. Toxins and chemicals are either produced from the immune system attacking itself or from direct ingestion of these particles. They can be absorbed so rapidly that the liver cannot break them down quickly enough. These various chemicals and byproducts can irritate nerve endings and affect cellular metabolism.

Sensitivities

I do not want to rule out the possibility that allergies can cause or contribute to muscle pain. I know that a sensitivity to calcium, magnesium or potassium can lead to muscle contraction and relaxation difficulties because malabsorption can create a deficiency in these key nutrients. Sensitivity to certain B vitamins can contribute as well, because B complex nourishes the nerves, which feed the muscles. Hyperexcitability in nerve functioning can cause improper signaling of nerve impulses leading to hypercontracted muscles. Sensitivities to common foods that are eaten on a regular basis can cause chronic muscle tightness and pain. Many patients in my practice have mentioned that their muscle pain seems to flare up in response to the ingestion of wheat.

Allergies affect the Chinese meridian system by causing either an excess or a deficiency of qi in specific meridians. This imbalance of qi will cause associated muscles for those meridians to either spasm with excess qi or become weak with deficient qi. Sensitivities to foods eaten on an occasional basis can cause intermittent muscle pain. That same food eaten on a regular basis can cause chronic pain. Sensitivities to any component of the Krebs cycle can lead to a deficiency of that component, which should not be ruled out as a possibility for muscle dysfunction.

Muscle dysfunction

Other factors can either cause or contribute to muscle dysfunction. A person may only feel slight muscle fatigue or soreness following exercise or exertion, may need a massage more often than normal, and may need to take extra magnesium daily to address the condition. The muscle endurance that they once had may have declined, or their muscles just feel tight. They may not recognize that there is a serious hidden problem, which is festering. These symptoms may have gradually crept up on them, and they think this is what normal feels like, because they have lost touch over the years with what feeling healthy was all about. Any of the above in combination, even at minute levels, can feed into these symptoms. This can progress to what is referred as full-blown fibromyalgia, which is a severe development of the above symptoms. Once people are at this stage, they are identified with a named "disease." The progression can begin slowly or be instantly triggered by many other factors. Many people develop full-blown fibromyalgia following a stressful time in their lives; this is due to the pathogen lying in a dormant state for years waiting for the opportunity to break out while the immune system is at its weakest point. The groundwork was laid and all that was needed was a trigger.

Mycoplasma infection

I believe that mycoplasma infection is the chief instigator of chronic muscle pain and inflammation. The best scenario for this is the Gulf War syndrome. *Mycoplasma fermentans* was found in at least 40 percent of the soldiers tested. Many had arthritis, fibromyalgia and chronic fatigue (Nicolson, March 25, 2000). *Mycoplasma penetrans* should also be on the high priority list. Again, any pathogen can be the culprit, as the bloodstream is an open highway for invasion. My research has shown mycoplasma infection, especially *Mycoplasma penetrans*, to be the most common causative agent. Once the source of this problem is rectified, which entails supporting the immune system in its removal, the body is then free from this systemic burden and the pain usually subsides. Muscle function returns to normal, and higher energy levels return.

I have seen many patients who were previously diagnosed with fibromyalgia and who are now free of muscle pain and fatigue because the root cause of their condition was addressed. Many times a patient's health is restored much more rapidly from fibromyalgia than any other chronic autoimmune conditions. The muscles are very resilient as damage is held to a minimum. I often joke with patients who come into my office with this condition. I say, "If you are going to be identified with an autoimmune disease, it is best to have been labeled with fibromyalgia."

Notes

Nicolson, Garth L., Ph.D. "VA Confirms Nicholson's Data on Chronic Infections in Gulf War Illness Patients," The Institute for Molecular Medicine, March 25, 2000. www.immed.org/illness/whatsnew/news00-3-25.html

References

Deadman, Peter and Mazin Al-Khafaji. *A Manual of Acupuncture*. Vista, California: Eastland Press, 1998.

Guthrie, Michael, R.PH. "Mycoplasmas: The Missing Link in Fatiguing Illness," *Alternative Medicine*, September 2001.

Nicolson, Garth L., Ph.D. "Autoimmune Illnesses and Degenerative Diseases," The Institute for Molecular Medicine, Accessed June 26, 2005. www.immed.org/illness/fatigue_autoimmune_illness_research.html

Nicolson, Garth L., Ph.D. "Chronic Fatigue Illnesses," The Institute for Molecular Medicine, Accessed June 26, 2005. www.immed.org/illness/infectious_disease_research.html

Nicolson, Garth L., Ph.D. "Chronic Infectious Diseases," The Institute for Molecular Medicine, Accessed June 26, 2005. www.immed.org/illness/fatigue_illness_research.html

Nicolson, Garth L., Ph.D. "VA Confirms Nicholson's Data on Chronic Infections in Gulf War Illness Patients," The Institute for Molecular Medicine, March 25, 2000. www.immed.org/illness/whatsnew/news00-3-25.html

Sinha, Gunjan. "Gulf War Illness: Psychological?" *Popular Science*, April 1999.

Chapter 38: Vaginal, Pelvic and Cervical Illnesses

Vaginitis refers to inflammation in the vaginal area. Pelvic inflammatory disease is inflammation located from the cervix to the uterus. Since they have similar origins and associated locations, I have grouped these illnesses together. Cervical dysplasia is an inflammatory pattern in the cervix that causes localized tissues to change forms.

Common infections

These infections are commonly caused by sexual intercourse. Since the woman is the receptor during sex, she runs a much higher risk of being infected. The more sexual partners a woman has had increase her chances of acquiring an infection. The vaginal area is a great place for microbes to multiply. One of the common pathogens that can reside in the vaginal area is *Candida albicans*, which is the cause of yeast infections. This usually comes about as a consequence of antibiotic therapy.

Gardnerella vaginalis, Trichomonas vaginalis, Haemophilus vaginalis, Mycoplasma hominis, Mycoplasma genitalium, Chlamydia trachomatis, Ureaplasma urealyticum, group B Streptococcus, human papillomavirus (HPV), *Neisseria gonorrhoeae,* the fungus lichen sclerosis or lichen planus, as well as some others, can locate in the vaginal area. The common symptoms are inflammation, tenderness, pain, dryness, foul odor and itching. Many women who harbor these pests may find it difficult to have intercourse due to the inflammation. These bugs can also be passed back to the male, which can cause many problems for him as well.

Candida albicans has become epidemic in our society due to the overuse of antibiotic therapy, steroids and birth control pills. *Candida albicans* loves moist dark places in which it can implant itself and flourish. It creates damp heat and allows other pathogens to flourish as it lowers immune function. Long-term or repeated antibiotic therapy is mostly responsible for creating this breeding ground and unhealthy environment. The damp heat and other pathogenic influences can set the stage for a chronic inflammatory pattern. The overuse of antibiotic therapy can lead to stronger forms of these bugs as they mutate in order to avoid being destroyed.

Traditional medicine does not usually test for all of the pathogens listed above. Many times test results will come back showing only a portion, or none of these pathogens present. *Mycoplasma hominis* is usually present in healthy vaginal tissue, but can become pathogenic once it invades the genital organs and tissues. *Ureaplasma urealyticum* is increasing in incidence. It is also a mycoplasma, as it often infects the kidneys as well. These bugs can also originate in the vaginal tract, mutate, grow in numbers and enter the bloodstream and/or lymph system. In these systems, they can easily travel to distant sites ending up in joints, organs or any other rest area along their journey.

Cervical dysplasia is usually caused by HPV, which is a wart virus. There are about thirty different variations of this virus. HPV 16 and 18 are the most common cause of cervical dysplasia. HPV is very slow moving and can lie dormant for years before manifesting. HPV has recently been implicated in cervical cancer. Most often carriers have no idea they are infected with it. Superficial signs are small raised bumps on the surface. A good gynecologist may be able to detect HPV from a pap smear.

Any chronic inflammatory condition in the pelvic, cervical or vaginal areas most often has one or more lingering pathogens underlying the named disease. Any bug has the ability to cause various symptoms including cysts and possibly cancer. Why would a virus such as HPV have the ability to cause cancer, but not any other pathogen?

The lymph system, which includes lymph nodes and vessels, are abundant in the groin area. This system and the bloodstream are excellent transport highways for traveling pathogens looking for a home. The pelvic, vaginal and cervical areas are the perfect environments in which to multiply. Any area with an inflammatory or chronic condition is almost sure to have a pathogenic influence driving the inflammation. It is so easy to infect and be infected by your partner, even if your partner seems healthy.

Partner treatment

I recently worked with a friend who is normally very healthy. She started a new relationship within the last year. Her male partner had no symptoms that would give her any concern. However, within a few months, she started to develop lower abdominal pain, which then moved more to the pelvic area. She often felt tired, unlike her normal self.

After examining her, I thought lingering pathogens may be underlying the symptoms. Once her immune system was able to overcome the offending invaders, her symptoms were completely eliminated and her energy and vitality returned. Her male partner's immune system also needed assistance. Luckily he was open to wanting to support her as well as himself, so that they both could be healthy together. Once you understand that transference of pathogens is highly likely with sexual intercourse, then wanting to protect your partner as well as yourself becomes a mutual and loving decision.

References

Hamza, Haizal, M.D. "Bacterial Infections and Pregnancy," eMedicine, Accessed June 8, 2005.
www.emedicine.com/med/topic3269.htm

Hansen, Eric, D.O. "Gardnerella," eMedicine, Accessed March 14, 2005.
www.emedicine.com/med/topic841.htm

Hiong U Go, Chi, M.D. "Escherichia Coli Infections," eMedicine, Accessed March 9, 2005.
www.emedicine.com/MED/topic734.htm

Lutwick, Larry, M.D. "Chlamydial Genitourinary Infections," eMedicine, Accessed March 14, 2005.
www.emedicine.com/MED/topic340.htm

Moore, Donnica, M.D. "Mycoplasma Hominis," DrDonnica.com, Accessed March 3, 2004.
www.drdonnica.com/faqs/00004901.htm

Snyder Sachs, Jessica. "Are Antibiotics Killing Us?" *Discover*, November 2005.

"What Is Lichen Sclerosus?" National Lichen Sclerosus Support Group, Accessed March 26, 2004.
www.lichensclerosus.org

Chapter 39: Urinary Tract/Bladder Disorders

Urinary tract and bladder disorders are usually caused from various types of bacteria that find their way into the urinary system. These conditions are more common in women than men due to the close proximity of the vagina to the urethral opening. Men can also acquire these disorders, but it is a bit more difficult due to the difference in anatomical structures. Sexual activity with multiple partners and low-immune function contribute greatly to increased incidence.

The role of pathogens

The most common bacteria are *E. coli, Klebsiella* and *Proteus vulgaris*. Two others are more likely to be acquired in hospital settings; they are *Pseudomonas* and *Enterobacter*. *Ureaplasma urealyticum* and *Mycoplasma genitalium*, which are both mycoplasmas, have been recognized by some in the scientific community as being leading role players in urinary tract disorders over the last few years. They seem to be showing up more and more as causative agents in urinary, kidney and bladder disorders. I believe these pathogens are easily transferred during sexual intercourse. *Trichomonas vaginalis* is a parasite that is also a common inhabitant of the urinary system. Other less common invaders can include *Candida albicans, Staphylococcus saprophyticus, group B Streptococcus, Enterococcus* and *Neisseria gonorrhoeae*. Many times there is more than one invader responsible for the symptoms.

Natural remedies

Cranberry juice is the most common nonprescription remedy used for clearing out the invading bacteria, and it seems to be fairly effective in some cases. Mannose is a sugar that has also shown to be of benefit. These two substances have the ability to pull the bacteria off the lining of the urinary tract and flush them out of the system.

Many supplement companies use herbal formulas that combine several herbs for a synergistic effect.

Chinese medicine uses various herbs, which help to reduce the heat and inflammation. Acupuncture can be very effective in helping to pull the heat out of the urinary tract.

All of the above can be fairly effective in reducing symptoms. When these methods fail and the bladder or kidney infection returns, then one or more of these lingering pathogens have probably rooted themselves into the lining of the urinary tract and/or bladder. Certain allergies and foods can also exacerbate the inflammation.

When these conditions become chronic in the urethra and/or kidney, then it is termed urethritis or simply called a particular form of kidney disease. If it lies within the bladder then it is called a bladder infection; when this infection becomes a chronic long-term condition, it causes the inability of the bladder to hold urine for any long period. This is because the bladder wall can become thick and inelastic due to the long-term inflammation, which forms scar tissue on the bladder's inner lining. Urination can become painful with increased frequency. A scarred bladder does not have the ability to expand and contract without re-tearing the old scar tissue. Thus the patient can be left with a permanent inflammatory condition much like arthritis within a joint. This condition may never permanently heal, even if the original offenders are removed. The condition is then called interstitial cystitis. See www.richbrightheart.com for nutritional and herbal support.

References

Emmons, Wesley W., M.D. "Urinary Tract Infection, Males," eMedicine, Accessed March 3, 2005.
www.emedicine.com/MED/topic2346.htm

Hiong U Go, Chi, M.D. "Escherichia Coli Infections," eMedicine, Accessed March 9, 2005.
www.emedicine.com/MED/topic734.htm

Nicolson, Garth L., Ph.D. "Chronic Infectious Diseases," The Institute for Molecular Medicine, Accessed June 26, 2005.
www.immed.org/illness/fatigue_illness_research.html

"What Is Urinary Tract Infection," Native Remedies, Accessed June 25, 2007.
www.nativeremedies.com/uti_clear_for_uti_bladder_infection.shtml

Chapter 40: Erectile Dysfunction/Low Libido

Most men do not want to talk with anyone about erectile dysfunction, especially with another guy. I have not had many men come into my practice complaining of this problem. Guess who I hear it from? That is right, the wife. The sales of Viagra and Cialis have skyrocketed in the last few years. Men in their thirties and forties are beginning to take these prescriptions to enhance performance. What a shame, as erectile dysfunction is a sure sign of their declining overall health.

Chinese medicine

Erectile dysfunction in Chinese medicine is due to poor kidney function. The Chinese diagnosis for this is called a jing or kidney deficiency. The kidneys control the sexual energy in both males and females. When kidney function drops, so does sexual energy. Think of being exhausted, "Do you really want to have sex?" Erectile dysfunction is a systemic problem in most cases. These are the same people who have to have their double latte in the morning just to function. Do you really need to ingest an artificial substance to do something that would be normal if your health was good?

The problem

This takes us back to Chapter 8 on Organ Degradation. Either external stress from a hectic life or internal stress from pathogenic invasion is causing energetic depletion. Either of these problems will weaken the kidneys and adrenals. Poor diet can also be a contributor with too many processed foods and not enough nutrition to fuel the system. Caffeine, smoking, alcohol and some medications, especially cholesterol-lowering statin drugs, will reduce testosterone levels. You can bet on having low libido with this type of lifestyle.

Pathogens can also get into the prostate and testicles and cause diminished sperm production and a general weakness in this area. Many men who have come into my office with a multitude of problems seem to gradually improve in this area without directly focusing on it. The positive effect happens when their system regains health by eliminating the pathogens and allergies, detoxifying the body, improving nutritional intake and receiving acupuncture treatments to eliminate the energetic blockage in the kidneys, thus supporting the overall body. These steps will give the kidneys and adrenals a welcome break, then sexual function can begin to return to normal.

Chapter 41: Thyroid Conditions

Thyroid conditions seem to be a major focus today in some clinicians' practices. Much has been written about why this important gland fails to function properly in a high percentage of individuals, especially after age forty. Some of the most recent information can shine a slightly different light on this subject.

Thyroid dysfunction

Many factors contribute to thyroid dysfunction. The most common dysfunction involves low thyroid output. Most people over forty years old fall into this category. Several key factors seem to play a role in improper thyroid functioning. These factors ultimately determine how the thyroid functions.

The adrenal glands play a major supporting role in thyroid functioning due to the secretion of certain hormones that influence thyroid function. The adrenals release cortisol as a response to stress. High cortisol levels seem to hinder pituitary output. Chronic stress and inflammation are suppressive to overall thyroid functioning due largely to the fact that they increase cortisol production by the adrenals. Cortisol is the body's own built-in anti-inflammatory hormone. The pituitary gland produces human growth hormone (HGH); a lack of this hormone can hinder hormone conversion in the thyroid. This is why it is more difficult to keep the weight off as we age due to reduced output of HGH from a poor functioning pituitary. Certain minerals and vitamins (such as iodine, selenium, zinc and vitamin A also play a supporting role in thyroid function.

Autoimmune thyroid conditions can also influence the thyroid by either causing an overactive or underactive gland. The immune system is attacking the thyroid causing inflammation and swelling to occur, much like it does in other areas of the body. Left unattended permanent damage can result. In Hashimoto's disease, the thyroid becomes underactive. Graves' disease is a result of an overactive thyroid. With Graves' disease, the thyroid eventually burns itself out resulting in a hypothyroid. Thyroid antibody testing can determine if this is taking place.

The role of pathogens and heavy metals

The most likely culprits that cause an autoimmune thyroid are pathogens and heavy metals. The lower neck area is greatly affected by adjacent anatomical sites. The thyroid is close to cervical lymph glands, as well as the mouth. We know that bacteria from the mouth can infect the lymph vessels in the neck or travel down into the heart. The lungs are also relatively close anatomically. These three areas can all harbor lingering pathogens. All it takes is one pathogenic strain to venture its way into the thyroid gland. Once there, these critters multiply and emit toxins. Inflammation, swelling and eventual damage becomes the effect as the immune system continues to attack, but fails to remove the cause. *Staphylococcus* and *Streptococcus* are common bacteria that tend to reside in these adjacent tissues. They should be primary suspects if thyroid problems occur. *Mycoplasma gallisepticum*, usually more common in chickens, could be the culprit as well. So many lingering pathogens are found in this area that potential invaders can be numerous.

Mercury or any other heavy metal that may be lurking in the mouth can descend into the thyroid and cause a similar immune response.

At some point with the confirmation of antibody response, you will be tagged with a named disease label such Hashimoto's disease or Graves' disease.

Symptoms and testing

Common symptoms of a low thyroid include fatigue, weight gain, depression, constipation, dry skin, sensitivity to cold, dry skin, cold hands and feet, facial edema and loss of hair both from the top of your head as well as the outside portion of the eyebrows. An overactive thyroid will produce weight loss, anxiety, nervousness, hyperactivity and heat intolerance.

Traditional lab testing focuses on the thyroid stimulating hormone (TSH) as being the primary way of determining how the thyroid is functioning. This hormone is produced in the pituitary gland. It is secreted when thyroxin (T4), a thyroid hormone, levels drop. TSH stimulates the production of T4 and another thyroid hormone, triiodothyronine (T3), within the thyroid gland with the help of iodine. That is the reason iodine is so vital to proper thyroid functioning.

When testing for TSH, a high output indicates that the thyroid is underactive, because it is trying to compensate for a lagging thyroid gland. Many clinicians will focus on this and only this marker in determining the thyroid function and the patient's protocol. As long as TSH levels are in the normal range then it is assumed that this gland is functioning well. This, however, is a shortsighted approach and clearly does not give enough information to determine the whole picture.

Most physicians then will place the patient on some type of thyroid medication in order to stimulate the thyroid to produce T4, which will help to lower TSH output. This may indeed lower TSH markers, but may or may not improve overall functioning of this vital gland. The conversion of T4 to T3 is a major factor that can greatly influence thyroid function. T3 is a much more active form than T4, and is primarily responsible for increased metabolism. This conversion cycle can be lacking, even in a person who shows normal TSH levels. It is referred to as deficient conversion. An enzyme 5'diodanase (5'D-1) supports this conversion process, which takes place in the liver, brain and kidneys. If this enzyme is deficient then inadequate conversion can occur.

Other factors besides human growth hormone can also influence this process. They include a possible sensitivity to the 5'D-1 enzyme, stress, some drugs and radiation. Cell phones and computers may be a factor, as any radiation to the head and neck area seem to be a contributing impact. Soy products have also been known for years to negatively affect this conversion cycle. Many Americans are now using soy as an alternative to milk due to allergies, phlegm production and the avoidance of hormones, steroids and antibiotics that are so prevalent in the dairy industry.

The role of minerals and chemicals

Minerals play a major role in the conversion of T4 to T3. Iodine is a key nutrient that seems to perform a main function in this conversion. Some practitioners think that iodine is needed only for the prevention of goiters. Therefore, if we have sufficient iodine in our intake, which we get mostly from table salt, then we have sufficient iodine for thyroid functioning and the prevention of goiters. However, others argue iodine has a more important role in the body.

One of the leading proponents of iodine is David Brownstein, M.D., who has written an intriguing book, *"Iodine: Why You Need It, Why You Can't Live Without It."* Last fall, I attended a class taught by an avid supporter of Dr. Brownstein's views on iodine.

I have taken several workshops over the last few years that were related to thyroid functioning. Although all the workshop presenters agreed that TSH testing is not an overall accurate assessment of thyroid functioning, they offered slightly different views on what is the best approach for supporting this gland.

Dr. Brownstein's book shines a whole different light on this valuable mineral. He thinks that iodine in proper proportions has a positive effect on thyroid functioning. Brownstein claims that many of his patients have benefited from supplementation, especially in the areas of increased energy levels, mental health and improved immune functioning. He also examines the negative effects that several common ingestants have on thyroid function. In the halogen family, they include: chlorine, used as a bleaching and disinfectant agent; bromine, used in baked goods, some medications and as a disinfectant for pools and hot tubs; and fluoride, used in toothpaste as well as our drinking water. These halogens seem to take up the binding sites located in the thyroid that should be reserved for iodine. This seems to hinder the gland's functioning, according to Dr. Brownstein. If what he says is true this information would be highly valuable in restoring a sluggish thyroid (Brownstein, 2006).

Actions to take

Iodine levels can be determined by testing, which is called an iodine-loading test. This test can show current body levels and then appropriate supplementation can be employed.

Always remember that a deficiency of iodine may be due to a sensitivity to it. If iodine is found to be a reactant then sensitivity repatterning should be used before supplementation takes place. See Chapter 10: Nutritional Sensitivities Equal Nutritional Deficiencies.

If you want to look further into more investigative testing methods, labs are available that can give you about a half dozen specific markers to provide you with more in-depth information on why your thyroid may not be functioning properly. With this information, you will be able to focus on areas of concern with supplementation, detoxification or pathogenic elimination.

Notes

Brownstein, David, M.D. *Iodine: Why You Need It, Why You Can't Live Without It.* West Bloomfield, Michigan: Medical Alternatives Press, 2006.

References

Sack, J. et al. "Binding of Thyrotropin to Selected Mycoplasma Species: Detection of Serum Antibodies Against a Specific Mycoplasma Membrane Antigen in Patients with Autoimmune Thyroid Disease," PubMed, Accessed October 31, 2006. www.ncbi.nlm.gov/entrez/query.fcgi?cmd=Retreive&db=PubMed&list_uids=2754 187&dopt=abstract

Chapter 42: Skin Conditions

Skin problems are usually categorized into various compartments, depending upon how the breakout appears. Psoriasis, scleroderma, dermatitis and eczema are the common skin conditions.

The problem

The first thing to understand about skin disorders is that even though they appear at the surface level of the body, rarely is the cause on the surface of the epidermis. These are usually deep-seated problems that are showing themselves outwardly. When you see an outbreak, it usually looks like some type of rash. This rash is red or pink in color. It shows an internal inflammatory pattern that has surfaced. What is underlying this surface representation is usually a response to a pathogen, allergen or toxin. The other possibility is a toxic liver that has created a lot of heat and toxins. Sometimes as toxins try to leave the body, they will appear as a rash, etc. Our skin is considered a system of the body that has cleansing properties. Putting a lotion or salve on the area may give temporary relief. However, this in no way addresses the cause of the underlying problem.

The role of pathogens

Staphylococcus is a common bacterium that tends to cause more skin problems in the head, face and neck area. I have seen breakouts several times in this area that I believe was due to staph infection. Once the immune system clears the *Staph* out, it usually clears up the external manifestation fairly quickly. I had a patient who was a carrier of *Strep*. Once his immune system was able to kick the *Strep* out, both the acne and the sore throat left simultaneously. Various fungi also are potential pathogenic causes.

Itching is also commonly caused by either pathogens or allergies. I see allergies as a huge component of itching. Histamine reactions caused by allergies can induce itching. Skin breakouts and itching in the genital area after sexual intercourse are usually due to the exchange of pathogens, which are being attacked by our immune system. When patients report to me that they usually get some type of rash or discharge after intercourse, this is the body's warning system going off. I once had a patient whose hands and feet were so red and scaled that she had to wear gloves all the time. They itched so badly that she was in constant misery. The underlying cause was lingering pathogens. Once her immune system was able to take charge and kick these critters out, the skin immediately started to improve.

Sensitivities

Allergies to a specific food eaten occasionally may cause intermittent episodes of itching and rashes, unless it is a food consumed on a regular basis such as wheat, corn or dairy that might cause the same symptoms consistently. Also basic nutrient allergies can be a causative factor because they are components of foods that we eat. An allergy to vitamin A, for instance, could cause a deficiency of that vitamin in your system. Vitamin A is a key nutrient for healthy skin.

Scleroderma

Scleroderma is a chronic condition of hardening of the skin that is under the autoimmune classification. When pathogens are present just below the skin level, the body's response to this is to cause a low-grade inflammatory condition. This process causes the body to send collagen to the area in order to buffer the inflammation. This contributes to the thickening of the skin in areas that are under attack. Mycoplasmas are highly indicated as causative agents in these conditions. The inflammatory process then does its thing, which causes the skin to become fibrotic in nature. The body is smart, so when some part is under stress, it has its own built in protective devices.

Diagnosis or cure

I once had a patient who came in with fairly severe rashes over her arms and hands. She had just come from a well-respected skin clinic in Seattle. She raved on about this wonderful specialist who was a highly regarded leader and lecturer in her field. This specialist was good at being able to classify her condition into a specific category. My new patient seemed impressed with the specialist, as she now definitely knew what her category of an effect was labeled. I asked her what the skin specialist said about the prognosis was for arresting it. She replied that the specialist really did not have any way of treating it, except using salves and creams to reduce the effects when it flared up, which she had already been doing with little improvement. I then pointedly asked what the actual value to her was for getting such an insightful diagnosis? She looked puzzled and said, "I am not sure, except that I have a name for it now." My point is that having a proper diagnosis for a condition is fine. Your specialist may indeed be the best at placing your symptoms into the right category. However, it carries little value to the patient, unless the specialist has a way of curing it. Can you imagine taking your car to a foreign car specialist, Antonio, and he brilliantly diagnoses the problem, but has no way to fix it? You would be outraged by this way of thinking. You would say, "What good does it do me, Antonio, if you can't fix it? Your diagnosis is absolutely worthless to me!"

References

Hitti, Miranda. "Experts Call for Worldwide Vigilance to Slow Methicillin-Resistant Staph's Rise," MedicalNet, June 21, 2006.
www.medicinenet.com/script/main/art.asp?articlekey=62615 - 38k

Tacoma-Pierce County Health Department and Spokane Regional Health Department. "Living with MRSA (Methicillin-Resistant Staphylococcus Aureus)," Fall 2004.

Chapter 43: Electromagnetic/Invisible Smog

Electromagnetic/invisible smog is a fairly new term that has come about in the last decade due to the progress we have made in many forms of technology, especially computers and cell phones. The use of this technology has gone far ahead of what we know about how it affects the body. There has been more than a trillion times increase in these frequencies over the last two decades. This type of pollution may already be, or surely will become, the greatest pollutant this planet has ever "not seen."

The problem

Why electromagnetic/invisible smog is so lethal has to do with its invisible nature. If we cannot see it, how can we gauge its effect? This is a big part of the problem. Pollution from autos can be seen miles away as well as smelled. Our senses, just like the sense of animals, were installed by our creator partly for protection. On the other hand, people can be in a closed room, smack in the middle of dense cloud of electromagnetic radiation, without seeing or smelling a thing. Does that mean it does not exist and has no physiological effect on us?

Many people remember that the tobacco manufacturers held back vital information on the chemical additives and effects from smoking that they purposely kept secret from the public for decades. Doctors once promoted cigarettes as being healthy and recommended that pregnant women smoke in order to keep their weight down. They also believed that diet had little to do with being healthy. I am not putting cell phones and other electromagnetic frequency devices in the same category as cigarettes or poor diet. However, considering our history of protecting people from tobacco and realizing that electromagnetic frequency may be a carcinogen of another kind, we should have concerns that little is known about the accumulative long-term effects that might develop. The damage to the body could be on par or even greater than what we now know about the effects of secondhand smoke and its effects on cancer, aging and lung disorders. The rapid growth and expansion in the electromagnetic frequency industry is mind-boggling. The constant exposure to these electromagnetic frequencies over time may be the largest biological experiment to date. We again get to be the rats that are being experimented on in this very real life research project.

Lessons from history

In addition to learning about the dangers of smoking cigarettes, we have had to figure out the dangers of: eating livestock which had been fed antibiotics, steroids and hormones, filling teeth with mercury, breathing polluted air, and eating fish loaded with mercury and other toxins.

This thinking took years to come about as technology, lack of information and the flow of money went ahead of potential health concerns. It usually takes about twenty years for us to learn from our ignorance. We may be in the dark ages once again, due to the lack of information on, or misinformation about, this emerging electromagnetic generation. The playing field has changed; convenience, technology and big business are going full throttle ahead once again, before knowing much of the potential consequences that may lay waiting.

Electromagnetic illness

Electromagnetic illness can show up in both acute and chronic forms. Some common acute symptoms from electromagnetic radiation include headaches, fatigue, dizziness, nausea, depression, insomnia, difficulty in concentrating and memory loss. These symptoms may only be short term, as they may decrease or totally disappear once the cause is removed. Possible long-term health risks may be at a deeper level that we are only beginning to understand. Cancer and other serious health problems are usually slow to manifest, as it takes years for them to show their ugly faces. It may take decades before all the facts are in, so we can properly unravel this data. Hopefully, we have learned enough from our past mistakes that convenience does not always equal positive long-term benefits to the most important area of our life, our health.

Cell phones, unfortunately, are not our only concern as a wave of new technology encompasses other contributive forces. Devices of concern include everything from hair dryers to computers. The future will also add other devices called silicon sensors. These microchips will be embedded in everything from bumpers to vacuum cleaners. The reason cell and cordless phones are so problematic has to do with their proximity to the body, especially the brain which is the key exposure area. The length of time during the exposure is another variable. The last key element is the total amount of electromagnetic exposure. For instance, using an electric blanket at night in conjunction with having a clock radio sitting by your head is considered high exposure, due to the length of time and close proximity to the body.

The proximity to the ear is even more dangerous. It allows electromagnetic radiation to penetrate into the ear and brain tissue and affect the DNA within this tissue. A two-minute phone call can alter electrical activity within the brain for two hours. This can cause something as minor as having difficulty in thinking. However, repeating this event over time may accelerate the growth of cancerous cells and affect the repair mechanisms that are innate within the body. The body responds to frequencies by causing cell membranes to harden. This affects the transmission of nutrients and waste products in and out of the cell. It also disrupts communication signaling across the cell membrane. This can down-regulate various receptors and their pathways within the membrane itself. It can have cascading affects throughout the system. There is also evidence of weakening of the blood-brain barrier when on the cell phone. This can allow toxins, proteins and pathogens to easily cross this barrier, thereby invading brain tissue. It can set the stage for various chronic brain disorders, including the formation of tumors and other forms of chronic inflammation that can eventually contribute to tissue destruction. Such exposures can then lead to brain cancer, Alzheimer's, Parkinson's and host of other conditions that seem to have an unspecified origin.

Again, inflammation is the effect of pathogens, unwanted proteins and toxins that are lodged in any tissue, especially the delicate tissues of the brain. The immune system will attack anywhere, including the brain. Blake Levitt, author of *Electromagnetic Fields: A Consumer's Guide to the Issues and How to Protect Ourselves*, stated, "A worse frequency could not have been chosen for human anatomy." The body has natural barriers that were set in place for a reason. We keep tinkering with nature and expect no adverse consequences (Levitt, 1995).

This radiation, called electromagnetic frequency or EMF, is similar to what microwave ovens put out. The only difference being that it is in smaller dosages compared to microwaves. Radiation being emitted by cell phones can be divided into two types.

The first is the near field radiation plume, which penetrates about six inches from the antenna. Lying next to the head allows this radiation to enter into the brain. When these frequencies are absorbed into the head, they are strong enough to cause neurological damage. If you carry your cell phone on your hip, it then penetrates the flat blood forming bones of the hip. This can cause a reduction in sperm count in males of up to 30 percent. The increase of heat to the brain is an indicator of the transference of radiation being absorbed into the brain. I noticed that my ear would get warm following a fifteen-minute cell phone conversation.

The second type of radiation we are absorbing is called far-field radiation. This produces more subtle effects that can be accumulative over time. Electromagnetic radiation has had rapid growth in the last decade, which comes from many sources, not just cell phones. These include microwave ovens, computers, hair dryers, television and radio waves, cordless phones, car tracking devices, electrical wiring, power lines and security and remote control devices, to name a few. Think about how many of these frequencies have been implemented or drastically increased in the past two decades. Growing up we had a black-and-white television with six or seven channels, radio, gas stove, refrigerator and rotary phone (Levitt, 1995).

All of these EMF frequencies interfere with the human electromagnetic biofield. Reading Chapter 2 on Energy Medicine gives a basis for this understanding. These perverse energies that we are constantly absorbing are in conflict with our own innate electromagnetic system. Remember that every cell in the body is controlled by its inherent electromagnetic vibration. Any disruption in the communication within the cell itself, or between other cells, can set up the right environment for illness. Immune and neurological functions can be especially vulnerable to these constant frequencies. This constant bombardment may not show up physiologically for years in terms of potential health risks. Remember Chapter 25 on Cardiovascular Disease and how chronic infection takes years to bring about coronary heart disease. These illnesses are slow-burning fuses, once the environment is ripe for development.

The younger the user, the higher the risk, as the developing brain is much more vulnerable (Carlo, 2001). The reason is the formation of the brain during its growth phase and the underdevelopment of the skull, which is much thinner. Children now start early with cell phones. My generation's first big step into adulthood came around the age of sixteen with passing a driver's exam and getting a license. Now this event has been replaced much earlier with getting your first cell phone. Kids equate cell phone use with growing up, so it is almost seen as a privilege or even an obligation to use it for hours on end, with the only restriction placed on it being the overage of minutes. A teenager uses a cell phone for an average of 2,600 minutes per month. By the year 2008, an estimated 40 percent of all children between age eight and eleven will have cell phones. You would not sit back and watch your twelve-year-old chain smoke, gorge himself on candy and soda pop or drink a six-pack of beer. After reading this chapter, would you still buy him a cell phone?

Research on electromagnetic radiation

What are some of the known risks and what have experts already concluded in the early stages of what we presently know about electromagnetic radiation?

The World Health Organization (WHO) has stated that electromagnetic smog is one of the fastest growing environmental influence. WHO has serious concerns about health effects, as the levels that will continue to rise as technology advances could interfere with the electrical currents of the human body. The International Agency for Research on Cancer has stated that this smog is a potential human carcinogen (Insight Journal, August 1, 2007).

The U.S. Environmental Protection Agency noted a 200-fold increase in radio frequencies and microwave fields from 1980 to 1999. Peter Franch, M.D., found that "cells are permanently damaged by cell phone frequencies." He stated that this damage can be inherited from generation to generation. Dr. Franch also found that the production of histamine, which triggers bronchial spasms, is nearly doubled after exposure to mobile phone transmissions. This may have something to do with a 25 percent increase in asthma in the metropolitan Sydney area (Thomas, July 6, 2006).

Neil Cherry, Ph.D., a biophysicist from Lincoln University in Christ Church, New Zealand, stated that there is a higher rate of cardiac problems from electromagnetic radiation. He also said that cell phone transmissions can alter mood by affecting the calcium, serotonin and hormone levels in your body. This can lead to rage, anger, violence, depression and suicide. He said, "There are sixty-six epidemiological studies showing that electromagnetic radiation across the spectrum increases brain tumors in human populations." Two of those studies looked at brain tumors from cell phones. Cherry also said, "Cancer takes ten to twenty years to manifest before we may see this curve show itself." According to professor Leif Salford, a neurologist, "After a two-minute conversation, a cell phone's digitized impulses disable the safety barrier that isolates the brain from destructive proteins and poisons in the blood." Salford said, "It seems that molecules such as proteins and toxins can pass out of the blood while the phone is switched on and enter the brain." He also stated that diseases such as MS and Alzheimer's are linked to proteins being found in the brain (Thomas, July 6, 2006).

Roger Coghill, Ph.D., a biophysicist, found that cell phone transmissions damage the ability of the white blood cells to ward off infectious disease by disrupting the immune system's electromagnetic communication (Thomas, July 6, 2006). Denis Henshaw, professor of Human Radiation Effects at Bristol University, estimated that electromagnetic smog causes some 9,000 cases of depression. Smog can even make you allergic to other electrical devices (Insight Journal, August 1, 2007).

George Carlo, Ph.D., author of the book, *Cell Phone: Invisible Hazards in the Wireless Age*, is a public health scientist who was initially hired by the Telecommunication Industry to coordinate wireless industry research on cell phone safety. He has overseen to date the most extensive research into wireless safety. Carlo headed a five-year, twenty-five-million-dollar industry-sponsored study on possible radiation hazards (Carlo, 2001).

"There is definite risk that the radiation plume that emanates from a cell phone antenna can cause cancer and other health problems," Carlo stated in his book. Carlo found that rare tumors on the outside of the brain are more than doubled among cell phone users, particularly on the right side of the head, which is where most people hold their phones. He told ABC's "20/20" that cell phones cause genetic damage that leads to cancer. ABC recommended "prudent avoidance" of cell phones after finding that every cell phone they lab-tested exceeded the Federal Communication Commission's standards for EMF absorption rates. Carlo also stated that the more one uses a cell phone the greater the cellular destruction and health risks. Experiments on captive animals show that cumulative DNA damage is passed on to succeeding generations. An Adelaide Hospital study found that B-cell lymphomas doubled in mice within eighteen months of a one-hour exposure to power densities experienced by cell phone users. Carlo has also pointed out that there was a 50 percent higher risk of getting an acoustic neuroma (a benign tumor of the auditory nerve) with cell phone users after six years, than for nonusers. Carlo's book is eye opening. The scientific research behind his statements help to unravel the big picture that is being overlooked or even hidden by the flow of technology and money (Carlo, 2001).

Here is some additional evidence that may give us an idea as to the impact that cell phones may be having on the public. Brain cancer rates in the United States have increased 20 percent and Australia has seen a 40 percent increase since the introduction of cell phones. More than 70 percent of the brain tumors are located under the ear. There are 30,000 to 50,000 new cases of brain and eye cancer each year worldwide attributed to cell phone usage according to *Epidemic Curve, Safe Wire Initiative*. British military scientists have discovered that cell phone transmissions disrupt the brain sites for memory and learning, causing forgetfulness and sudden confusion. The U.S. Department of Energy found that using a cell phone severely impairs memory and reaction times. It also found that hands-free mobile speakerphones cause even more crashes because they typically emit ten-times more brainwave interference than hand held units.

Cell phones emit varying amounts of radiation. The lower the signal bar, the higher the exposure. Exposure at one bar is a thousand times greater than at four bars. Power up time, which happens within the first minute, is when you get the highest exposure. Handsets have a cord that contains a copper wire that acts as an antenna. This antenna picks up the EMF not only from your cell phone, but anything emitting EMF from the environment. Cordless phones are no better. The base unit acts as a cell phone tower for the handheld unit. In Germany and London, you get heavy fines for talking on your cell phone and driving. These two countries believe that the concerns are not primarily due to cell phone distraction, as much as it has to do with the adverse effects that cell phones have on brainwave patterns. Response time is similar to someone who is drinking.

Much like how we now view secondhand smoke, ten to twenty years from now we will hopefully have all the facts and data compiled on illnesses that EMFs cause. Until then, the jury is out. At some point, we might be saying to each other, "I cannot believe that we used cell phones and other electromagnetic frequency devices back at the turn of century, without any protection. What were we thinking back then?"

Protection from EMFs

We currently protect ourselves from secondhand smoke. Similarly, we need to develop ways now that can protect ourselves from electromagnetic radiation. I believe that these phones and other frequency emitting devices do have an impact on our body systems that may or may not give us immediate symptoms. However, the long-term effects may not show up for years. Many people who smoke cigarettes started early on and did not see any symptoms until their forties. A morning cough was the first sign that damage was increasing. Lung problems, heart disease, premature aging and cancer were just a matter of time. Poor diet also will take years to manifest illness at a cellular level. Many people who have pathogen-related illnesses, such as cardiovascular disease, arthritis and fibromyalgia, had few signs or symptoms until they reached their thirties and forties. In most cases, their initial low-grade infection started years earlier, unseen without symptoms. However, with time and the progressive weakening of their system, the chronic infection eventually took over their entire body, producing joint, muscle, vascular and systemic inflammation. If you have read up to this chapter, then you understand the relationship of chronic, low-grade inflammation to gradual tissue damage.

I personally have had a problem with my left ear after using a cell phone on that side. It happened after only three months of moderate volume usage. I acquired an acute sinus infection, which my immune system was able to quickly eliminate. However, the bacterium found its way from my sinus cavities into my left ear. It feels like there is fluid in the ear or something crawling around in it at times. I believe that my immune system was compromised on that side, which just happens to be the same side that I hold my cell phone on. This is probably why my immune system was not able to remove the bug. I have never had an ear problem in my life prior to this. The pathogenic invasion of my ear was during the same period of time that I suddenly had an increase of cell phone usage. I do not believe that this was a coincidence.

I now have protection on my cell phone and cordless phones with a disc that sticks on their surfaces. I also wear a pendant that helps protect my body from both local- and far-field exposure as well. The same discs are on both my laptop and home computer. In my computer room, I have a small unit that plugs into the wall, which helps to minimize the electromagnetic frequencies in that room, as I spend significant amounts of time on my computer. I definitely can tell a difference in how I feel now that I have these protective devices in place. I want to minimize my exposure as much as possible. I believe these small changes will make a huge difference both in the short term, as well as protecting myself from any long-term potential risk factors. Had I been using a protective device prior to my increased cell phone usage, I probably would not have developed the ear problem. I think that it would be very difficult to give up some of these conveniences for many people, including myself. My own research and personal ear experience have made me more aware and led me to believe that protection is next best to abstinence. Have we not heard this somewhere before?

Notes

Carlo, George, Ph.D., and Martin Schram. *Cell Phones: Invisible Hazards in the Wireless Age*. New York: Carroll and Graf Publishers, 2001.

Levitt, Blake. *Electromagnetic Fields: A Consumer's Guide to the Issues and How to Protect Ourselves*. San Diego, California: Harcourt, Brace and Company, 1995.

"Modern Gadgets Linked to Depression, Cancer, Miscarriages," Insight Journal, Accessed August 1, 2007.
www.anxiety-and-depression-solutions.com/articles/News/05100gadgets.php

Thomas, Will. "Grave Cell Phone Dangers Revealed," July 6, 2006.

campaignfortruth.com/Eclub/210305/CTM%20-%20phone%20dangers%20revealed.htm

References

Fosburg, Michael. "Health Effects of Electromagnetic Radiation," *Total Health*, Vol. 28, No. 1, April/May 2006.

Michrowski, Andrew, Ph.D. "New Problems With Cell Phones," The Planetary Association for Clean Energy Inc., November 27, 2005.

Ridley, Kim. "Wake-Up Call," *Ode*, December 2006.

Sellman, Sherrill, N.D. "A Deadly Obsession: Hooked on Cell Phones," *Total Health*, Vol. 27, No. 1, 2005.

Chapter 44: Effective Therapies

Naturopathy

Naturopathic physicians are licensed in many states and can give a person a natural approach to many illnesses using supplements, herbs and other methods. They are considered primary care physicians in some states.

Acupuncture

Acupuncture is a three-thousand-year-old therapy that is mostly known in this country for pain relief. However, it is as effective for many common conditions such as digestive problems, depression, fatigue, gynecologic conditions and injury rehabilitation, to name a few. Acupuncture and Chinese herbs together have proven to be an effective therapy for many other acute and chronic problems. Acupuncture will help speed up the healing process in any condition, as well as be great adjunctive therapy to any other modality.

Chiropractic

Chiropractic doctors help the body's nervous system to be free of nerve blockages allowing the body to function at optimum levels. This can be very effective for joint related problems, as well as overall health. There are numerous forms of chiropractic medicine.

Massage therapy

Massage therapy is very effective for pain and relaxation. Massage is also a great rehabilitative therapy following injuries of all types, especially auto accidents and sports injuries. There are many spin-offs from massage such as Rolfing and Soma, which focus more on the fascia and structure, working from the feet upward.

Energetic medicine

Energetic medicine is a broad term for various types of therapies that can either temporarily or in some cases permanently change energetic patterns in the body. (See Chapter 2: Energy Medicine.)

Homeopathic medicine

Homeopathic medicine is also considered an energy therapy that works much like a vaccine, using highly diluted frequencies of a substance. Taking this will stimulate specific immune functions. This is further covered in Chapter 2 on Energy Medicine.

Emotional healing

Emotional healing can come in many forms. There are forms of acupuncture, chiropractic, homeopathic and energy medicine that incorporate emotional techniques or philosophy into their practice. Some therapists use energy-based techniques as an adjunct to other therapies that they use within their gamut of tools. (See Chapter 2: Energy Medicine.) These techniques are quite powerful in terms of dealing with root issues.

Applied kinesiology

Applied kinesiology has been around since the 1980s. Some of the most innovative and powerful techniques have been developed from it. Muscle testing gives the practitioner a way in which she can access information from the body that is fast and many times very accurate. This information can open up the doorway to what is behind the disease process. Muscle testing can be quicker, more accurate and more encompassing than lab testing in many ways. Numerous therapies now use muscle testing within the confines of a specific technique. New forms are sprouting up all over the world.

Chiropractors, acupuncturists, mental health therapists and many other health practitioners use kinesiology to the patient's advantage. Kinesiology is not considered scientifically based; therefore, it is not taught in most alternative medicine schools. Some within the alternative community are even skeptical and do not understand the potential it can have in the right hands. However, if a person seeks out a doctor or practitioner who uses muscle testing in her practice, it is prudent that the patient work with an experienced practitioner who comes with high recommendations as testing can be somewhat subjective. This is even more important with an inexperienced practitioner.

Iridology

Iridology is a way of seeing disease patterns within the eyes. There are some well-trained iridologists in this country. This tool is mainly used for evaluation by seeing discrepancies within the eye itself. This is not a healing tool, but a way to diagnosis conditions.

Effective therapies

These are some of the broad base of therapies that are both established and effective. There are many other therapies not described in this book that have great potential and effectiveness.

References

Cutler, Ellen W., D.C. *Winning the War Against Asthma and Allergies: A Drug-Free Cure for Asthma and Allergy Sufferers.* Albany, New York: Delmar Publishers, 1998.

Deadman, Peter and Mazin Al-Khafaji. *A Manual of Acupuncture.* Vista, California: Eastland Press, 1998.

Giovanni, Maciocia. *The Practice of Chinese Medicine: The Treatment of Diseases With Acupuncture and Chinese Herbs.* London: Churchill Livingstone, 1994.

Lipton, Bruce, Ph.D. "The Wisdom of Your Cells," *Light of Consciousness*, Spring 2007.

Oschman, James L., Ph.D. *Energy Medicine: The Scientific Basis.* London: Churchill Livingstone, 2000.

Watson, Brenda, N.D., C.T. *Renew Your Life: Improved Digestion and Detoxification.* Clearwater, Florida: Renew Life Press and Information Services, 2002.

Conclusion

I wish all people were aware of how the disease progress unfolds. They would have a choice to do something about it or stay sick. Why is not more of this information readily available? It is tragic that so many people suffer, and will continue to do so because of lack of awareness. People must ultimately take their health into their own hands and become their own advocate. Knowledge is power in any business and a person's health is crucial. If people do not decide what is best for their life and health status, they will be subject to the way an institution determines how their disease process is to be handled. This often times is not in their favor, as big money comes into the picture. Our medical system spends far too much money on "disease management" rather than looking for a cure. Many people are starting to see that patchwork medicine is not the answer.

Our health care system

We need to ultimately take a hard look at how and why our healthcare system is portrayed in the media in the way it is; who profits and who loses? Why does the media mostly ignore alternative medicine and place the spotlight on drugs and surgery as the primary way health care is to be viewed? If people have only seen traditional medical experts, they may be surprised to find that there is a whole world out there with many safe and effective methods for healing whatever disease process that they have been labeled with.

I am not advocating that we should exclude traditional medical professionals from our team. We need traditional doctors for emergency medicine as well as in certain other areas that complement the overall health team. If a particular medical doctor is unwilling to cooperate in a person's healing process, the patient may want to fire the doctor and hire one that will. More and more traditional doctors are also starting to wake up and realize that their patients, for the most part, are not getting any better with the tools they were given. The medical doctor of the future will work in conjunction with other health experts for the ultimate betterment of the patient. Unfortunately, the resistance for this change to fully take place comes from the very schools and institutions that have an enormous vested interest in keeping things the way they are. There is huge money in illness and disease management.

Information available

People must first have an open mind and an interest of gaining knowledge about their disorder. Researching and studying as many avenues as possible will give them the proper foundation to decide the most accurate type of healing method to alleviate their suffering. This may be in the form of alternative or traditional medicine, acupuncture, chiropractic, naturopathic medicine or massage therapy. These are viable and safe ways to incorporate various healing modalities into your health care.

The root cause

Always remember that if the treatment selected does not address the root cause, or at least have a means at working towards that goal, then that particular method should be questioned. Most people would never take their car to a mechanic and allow him to make drastic repairs to the car without questioning the mechanic and the reasoning behind the diagnosis. Most people have a better understanding of how their car functions than their own body. Therefore, they feel empowered when they question the mechanic, but feel reluctant to question their medical expert. Some medical doctors use fear-based statements in order to motivate the patient to act quickly in the direction the doctor wants to take them. I cannot count the number of patients who have come into my office upset because of something a doctor has told them about their condition. Many times they are told that something bad will happen unless they take drastic action immediately such as surgery or an experimental drug.

When people are told they have a disease of some type and are unfamiliar with the background of that illness and the options that may be available, it is easy to allow any medical practitioner or a person who has a vested interest in persuading them over to their way of thinking. Bad decisions at crucial times due to lack of awareness and fear-based motivation by the perceived medical authority can be critical, not only to the patient's recovery, but to her very life as well.

Alternative therapies

Read, research, use the Internet and talk with various types of healers and health care providers about their knowledge and success with a problem or condition you may be experiencing. Most medical doctors have very little knowledge of other methods that do not involve drugs and surgery. Their opinion is often swayed in this direction. The chef at one restaurant will not tell customers about the wonderful menu that her competitor has down the road, unless she wants to lose business.

Usually a week or two is all it takes to access proper information. When people have gained enough background and insight to the information and feel comfortable with a certain method, then the healing process has a much better chance for success. This process may incorporate a host of healers that have specialties in certain areas. Illness can be complex, so an aware and knowledgeable patient can have a team of practitioners and doctors that he feels comfortable with, knowing that each has strengths and weaknesses. Also, when people have the full trust in each person on their wellness team, they know that their goals are in alignment with those of the practitioner.

The desire of the practitioner for the wellness of the patient should be as much a concern to the practitioner as it is to the patient. This will assist people in getting well with much less dependence in the future on the practitioner. This can only happen when the root causes of illness are addressed. Utilizing the strengths of each individual practitioner along with self-education may be the best approach toward long-term wellness.

References

Abramson, John, M.D. *Overdosed America: The Broken Promise of American Medicine*. New York: Harper Perennial, 2005.

Deadman, Peter and Mazin Al-Khafaji. *A Manual of Acupuncture*. Vista, California: Eastland Press, 1998.

Garritano, Joanna, M.D. "U.S. Health Care Puts Profit Over People," *Seattle Post-Intelligencer*, January 10, 2007.

Moynihan, Ray and Alan Cassels. *Selling Sickness: How the World's Biggest Pharmaceutical Companies Are Turning Us All Into Patients*. New York: Nation Books, 2005.

Appendix: Testimonials From Patients

Testimonial No. 1

I had fibromyalgia and arthritis for many years and had appointments with doctors and specialists, epidermal injections, and many tests to try and get my body back to a normal and active life. I was getting depressed and my energy level was slowly going down due to my illnesses that were effecting my body.

In spring of 2006, I came to know Rich Brightheart from a friend who had been going to him for many of the same reasons as myself. I was encouraged about what she had told me about her visits to Rich. I had found the solution to my health problem. Because of Rich's knowledge and abilities, I am pain free. I feel that my energy level is above normal for my age. I thank God every day for God's blessing.

Nancy F., August 2006

Testimonial No. 2

Thanks to two of my daughters, I was introduced to Richard and his expertise. I am seventy-three years of age and, as you can imagine, very apprehensive about these treatments my daughters were urging me to get.

I was hooked on my first visit when Richard explained to me that he worked on the cause of an illness, not merely the symptoms. I had been suffering for a year with what doctors termed plantar fasciitis in my heel. After two weeks of treatment by Richard, my foot is no longer troubling me. I am now into my second week of treatment for inflammation and pain in my joints, which doctors called rheumatoid arthritis. I am already feeling the positive results of that.

I hope to be able to continue on with Richard to clear other problems, which I have been trying to control with medications. My hope is that someday insurance companies will recognize this method of dealing with diseases and illnesses in general so that more people can benefit.

Thank you, Richard.

Carla C., 2006

Testimonial No. 3

Rich worked on my thyroid in July of 2006. I was told I had very little if any activity in my thyroid in 1992 and was put on synthroid medication. I asked Rich to work on my thyroid. I felt more energy and better health-wise after just four to five treatments.

About the seventh treatment, I woke up in the middle of the night with my thyroid throbbing, no pain. It was like my thyroid had been awakened. Rich finished the treatments and I feel great. I am even finally being able to lose weight. It feels so good to be on the healing path.

Thank you, Rich.

Sharon K., 2006

Testimonial No. 4

I am writing with the skeptic in mind. I will be 50 this year, and I think that there will probably always be some sort of ache or pain. However, when something awakens me out of sleeping, it's time to address the issue. I have somewhat lost my faith in traditional institutions. My hip is much better. One night upon exiting my vehicle, I tried to limp as I always limp for twenty feet or so, wrong. No pain.

There was an issue with my wrist, a lump growing and pain. It's gone. Work with Rich. If I have more issues, I will hunt him down.

Heather, October 2005

Testimonial No. 5

Several years ago, I was diagnosed with acid reflux. Three years ago my stomach started hurting, and I could find no relief. I consulted a gastroenterologist who put me through a variety of tests. He then put me on a medication (Prevacid), which I took for three years. Not only was it very expensive, but I didn't like being on medication for my lifetime.

I came to Rich for treatments and was delighted that his work relieved the stomach ailment and the need for Prevacid. I have been pain free for three months. And I own it all to Rich's expertise.

Carla C., 2006

Testimonial No. 6

It has been a month since my treatments ended, and I can truly say they have changed my life. The most significant change for me has been your successful treatment of my decades-long extreme photosensitivity to the sun.

While numerous doctors and specialists have been mystified by this for years, you determined that I was sensitive to both Vitamin D and radiation and then repatterned my body to not react to those substances. I am so grateful to you for giving me the freedom to enjoy sunshine! As a result, I am having a fabulous summer and am looking forward to future vacations in sunny climates.

In reviewing my journal entries for the month I spent in Olympia, I am reminded of how many of my symptoms have disappeared altogether – some of which I sought treatment for and some I didn't mention to you.

One of those symptoms I didn't mention, a sense of "tipping" to the right, I had attributed to a motor vehicle accident and resulting multiple fractures to my left leg. To my surprise and delight, that balance issue has disappeared.

My blood pressure has also stabilized—another positive outcome of the treatments!

Overall, so many things have improved or vanished that, were it not for my journal, I wouldn't even remember what the original symptoms were because I feel so healthy.

Thank you so much, Rich, for giving me this gift of health.

Linda G., 2008

Testimonial No. 7

I was treated in June and July of 2002. Rich cleared me of many things that I had not known were a problem. In the years since then, I realized that I no longer awoke in the night with my arms asleep and giving me pain. I feel sure that Rich has been a big reason I am a healthy, active and pain free seventy-six year old.

Margaret H., 2002

Testimonial No. 8

I had contracted the virus that causes Bell's palsy. This was very painful and my doctor had said that there was nothing that she could do. It could last for months and still recur.

After two treatments with Rich the pain was gone. The same with a mouth infection. It had spread to my teeth till there was no place in which to bite down on. After two treatments, the pain was gone, and it has not returned.

Another thing Rich does is allergy repatterning. Calcium is one example. For years, my bone density had been decreasing. I tried taking osteoporosis medication, but the side effects were severe. Six months after correcting my calcium allergy my bone density increased 4 percent.

The most important change was neurological. I was diagnosed with bipolar disorder, chronic depression and anxiety attacks. For years, I tried everything I could to help myself. I tried psychiatric drugs, anticonvulsive drugs, several sleeping pills, muscle relaxants and every type of antidepressants. The side effects kept me very sick, and I only slept four to five hours per night. Finally, I was put on a mood stabilizer that I could tolerate. It moderated my symptoms but didn't get rid of them.

Treating this took a lot longer than the other problems. Pathogens and allergies that interfered with neurotransmitter and brain chemical imbalances. I am no longer depressed or anxious. I sleep fine. I feel happy. I am happy doing things I care about every day.

L.S., 2006

Testimonial No. 9

When I first came to you in February of this year, I was at the end of what allopathic medicine could do for me, and at the end of my rope. I was continually fighting sinus and ear infections to no avail. I realized that if I was going to survive on this planet, in this body, that I needed to try alternative medicine.

It's amazing looking back a few months ago to realize how sick I was, knowing how well I feel today physically and emotionally after undergoing treatments. Through the use of Sensitivity Response Repatterning my allergies have been significantly reduced. My foggy thinking has been cleared, and I am able to concentrate for the first time in a long time. The day I could actually breathe again through my nose was absolutely spectacular! I appreciate that you have the wisdom and expertise to know how to balance the whole person, rather than simply treating a symptom as conventional doctors do.

Thank you for taking the time to ferret out the many substances my body could not absorb such as calcium, serotonin, and many vitamins and minerals that kept me from experiencing the joy of life. I also had soft tissue pain in my upper neck, shoulder blade and pain in my low back from a previous injury. After completing this series of treatments, the inflammation in my body has been seriously reduced, and I have a sense of well-being.

This work is profound; there is simply no other way to put it. I encourage anyone considering treatment with you to do so. There's really nothing to lose and everything to gain, most of all your health and well-being. I am grateful to you for the path you have walked in order to become capable, caring and the remarkable healer that you are today.

Julia, September 2003

Testimonial No. 10

I began my clearing experience in 2004. I had a severe reaction/allergy to vitamin C, which caused immediate diarrhea when ingested. It was cleared in one treatment and now I take 1000 mg of vitamin C every morning. My biggest clearing occurred in the spring of this year. I awoke one morning and wondered if I was dying! I could barely move. Complete loss of strength and extreme tiredness.

I managed to get to Rich and his office. After one treatment, I was much better, and after a total of seven or eight treatments, I was cured. God bless Rich.

Betty S., 2007

Testimonial No. 11

In spring of 1997, I became quite ill. I was exhausted, even though I slept twelve to fourteen hours a day. I had extreme tendonitis in both arms and severe pain throughout my upper body. I constantly dealt with near pneumonia respiratory infections. I was diagnosed with fibromyalgia, chronic fatigue and extreme tendonitis and ordered to stop work and think about disability. Well, I did not think that was wise, but asked my dean to assist me in reducing my workload.

The first few months I tried many different therapies to reduce my pain. I used acupuncture, massage therapy, relaxation techniques, and the doctor put me on Prozac. I felt better by the fall of 1997 and could work a normal day. However, I still slept more than twelve hours a day and had constant pain. My social life was nonexistent as all my energy went toward work and the daily routine of living.

In fall of 2001, I was referred by another therapist to Rich Brightheart. I began treatment right after 9/11, and saw Rich several times a week for about six months. In three months, the fibromyalgia pain was nearly gone. My energy began to come back and within six months I was feeling so much better. Within a year I had renewed energy and was living an active life. Today I am healthy and have tremendous energy for my life. I have had no reoccurring pain or pneumonia in six years. Rich Brightheart healed me and I have referred many people to him.

Kate, 2007

Testimonial No. 12

Until I went to see Rich Brightheart, my left arm was so sore I could hardly raise it to put on my coat or even put a shirt on over my head. I also had low energy and had trouble concentrating. I had gone to traditional, Western medicine practitioners and tried some physical therapy. That was a waste of time. I tried exercises my naturopath gave me. That also didn't help. I did yoga stretches and that didn't help either. I took lots of supplements and did three years of acupuncture, and that only made a slight difference in pain level.

Finally, I found Rich and within a few months the range of motion in my arm was radically different and the pain was gone. I felt more energy and mental clarity. The concept of lingering pathogens had never even occurred to me or any other practitioner I worked with. After a few months of regular treatments my arm was perfectly fine. I even forgot it ever was a problem. I have Rich to thank for that.

Maureen

Testimonial No. 13

I came to Rich because I was suffering from MS. I had lost my ability to walk on my own. I was using a cane and walking slowly. Rich was referred to me by my friends who had come to him for treatments. Rich tested me for sensitivities and found I was sensitive to many of the supplements I was taking. He found I had indicators that may be causing or contributing to my MS symptoms.

Rich began treating me four times week with acupuncture. After just over one week, I was able to walk on my own, and I put the cane away. Rich continued to treat me for a month and each day I was better than the last. He has now completed my treatments but continues to monitor my supplement schedule. I would recommend Rich to anyone and let him see what he can do for you.

Mike E.

Testimonial No. 14

At the end of 2002, I found myself living in a nightmare. I was in a bizarre medical accident at the medical clinic where I worked. Because of it, I not only lost my job and my profession for nearly thirty years, it also left me in a state of constant pain. I found myself on the receiving end of the healthcare system with an unusual ailment. I soon found myself fighting an uphill battle. Most doctors do not have much experience with electrical shock. They would take a look at me and when they saw no physical burns or lost limbs, they would conclude that the symptoms I was having were "all in my head."

I was plagued with crazy pains in my muscles and bones, had headaches and migraines and experienced terrible depression. For almost six years, I have gone through the motions of living. I have seen more than thirty medical doctors in many specialties, some from as far away as Chicago. When I came to Rich, I was surely at the end of my rope.

After Rich began treating me, changes came on slowly at first, then I progressively got better. I've been hiding how bad things were for so long, it was a wonderful surprise to realize that I do not have to "act" anymore and that I am okay. Finally, I am moving forward with my life again.

Thank you, Rich, for my improved health and giving me my life back. My family and friends thank you. I will be eternally grateful.

Sharyn, September 2008

Testimonial No. 15

I brought my daughter Ariana, age fourteen, to Rich for ten sessions. She had a mysterious virus, with symptoms of morning nausea and vomiting. The previous year, she was in the emergency room three times. She had overall malaise and felt ill every morning for more than two months. We came to Rich as a last hope. During her treatments, Ariana got a cold, which normally would have put her out for over a week. Rich treated her with acupuncture and within two days she was fine.

In conclusion, Ariana's nausea, vomiting and dizziness are completely gone. She is feeling great and full of energy. My husband and I are both amazed and pleased. We will return to you in the future.

Nicki R.

Testimonial No. 16

Destiny, my daughter, is now sixteen and has been dealing with pain throughout her body for most of her life. We have taken her to doctors for years for the pain in her legs, head and stomach. Western medicine has failed her. She has low thyroid, gluten intolerance, multiple food allergies, fibromyalgia and who knows what else. She sleeps but has no energy. Since coming to Rich, we've seen such an improvement in Destiny. The biggest testimony is that she gladly comes for her treatments because she knows they are making a difference.

Thank you.

Valarie, September 29, 2009

I have hurt for as long as I can remember. It was such a constant feeling I thought it was normal. As I got older, everyone thought I was faking it. After awhile I started to believe them. My mom took me to countless doctors who gave me a silly excuse or told me that there was nothing wrong or they could not fix it. I had this false sense of hopelessness for so long.

Ever since I have been going to Rich, the pain is gone. It was constant for so long, I was numb to it. I am not irritable now, and I feel better. I have more energy and sleep through the night.

We have been waiting for an answer for so long, and now I'll finally be able to be normal, just one in a crowd. Someone who does not have to make a big deal out of every time she eats because I will get sick. I can eat ice cream. My favorite. I can jump on the trampoline for more than five minutes without getting tired. I can just live life. I really do not know how to put into words how grateful I am. I feel like God will take care of that just like he takes care of me.

Destiny

Testimonial No. 17

Here are the positive things I have experienced as a result of your work. I am forever grateful.

- My emotional well-being has improved. It has improved so much. I use to cry up to three or four times a week for long periods. Now I am not. Even during hormonal times of the month, I am way better emotionally. I still get angry, irritable and a little bitchy, but I am so much better. There is no comparison.
- My libido has improved greatly.
- My life force is so much stronger. I really feel strong and powerful, not because I am saying that I am. I really feel it.
- I am able to take on more responsibilities, do more and have fun doing it.

- I am so much more happy, enjoying life and laughing more.
- I am not as depressed as I was. There is no comparison.
- My eyes are shining, and I feel beautiful. There is much more life in my eyes.
- My mental functioning has greatly improved. I am not spacey much anymore.
- I am quickly more present, and it is easier to stay present these days. I feel like I have higher functioning. I can take in more information and understand it more readily. I am more relaxed. I do not feel as serious or in survival mode as I use to.
- My complexion is way better.
- My overall health, and my immune system, is better, a lot better.
- I feel safe in the world.

I am sure I could go on but enough for now. Thank you so much, Rich. You are a special man. I look forward to seeing you more in the near future for acupuncture.

Shannon

Index

Lyme disease 1, 79, 81, 91, 127, 134, 135, 136, 140, 141, 142, 143, 144, 145, 146, 148, 149, 150, 151, 152, 153, 156, 168, 192, 198
Lyme pathogen 147
Lyme symptoms 141, 150
lymph system 19, 40, 65, 147, 206, 207
lymphatic overload 144, 147
lymphatic system 40, 144, 161, 202
macular degeneration 46, 53, 105, 146
magnesium 21, 145, 168, 202, 203, 204
magnets 11
mangoes 47, 49
massage therapy 133, 228
melatonin 166
Meniere's disease 149, 183
meningeal tissue 132
meningitis 83, 132, 133, 136
meningitis, children 137
mental impairment *See* statin drugs
mental retardation 89
mercury 37, 66, 137, 145, 157, 158, 164, 198, 213, 220
mercury fillings 66, 145
mercury toxicity 66
Metabolic syndrome 160, 161
metabolism 50
methicillin-resistant Staphylococcus aureus (MRSA) 177
methylation detoxification 147
microflora 68
microglia cells 159
microorganism 79
mitochondria 50, 97
mononucleosis 81
mood swing 146
Moraxella catarrhalis 178

multi-pathogenic communities 145
multiple pathogenic factor 193
multiple sclerosis 1, 84, 132, 134, 148, 150, 159, 167
muramic acid 92
muscle dysfunction 204
muscle pain 30, 116, 145, 148, 198, 202, 203, 204, 205
muscle weakness 119
mycobacteria 1, 93, 198
  Corynebacteria 95
  Corynebacterium diphtheriae 95
  Leptospira 137
  Moraxella catarrhalis 180, 184
  Mycobacterium avium complex 95
  Mycobacterium avium intracellulare 95, 96
  Mycobacterium tuberculosis 95, 137
  Nocardia 95, 137
mycoplasma 1, 79, 81, 83, 87, 90, 91, 93, 96, 97, 98, 99, 100, 101, 113, 127, 136, 143, 145, 148, 149, 150, 151, 152, 156, 168, 169, 172, 173, 180, 184, 192, 194, 197, 198, 200, 204, 205, 206, 208, 209, 213, 215
  infection 91, 99, 136, 193, 204
  Mycoplasma fermentans 81, 90, 98, 136, 180, 184, 197
  Mycoplasma genitalium 90, 98, 206, 209
  Mycoplasma hominis 99, 206
  Mycoplasma incognitus 98, 157
  Mycoplasma penetrans 99
  Mycoplasma pneumoniae 98, 172, 173
  Mycoplasma salivarium 98
  Ureaplasma urealyticum 99, 206, 209
mycotoxin 102, 103, 143, 144
myelin sheath 134

About the Author

With more than thirty years of combined experience as a doctor of oriental medicine (acupuncturist) and licensed massage therapist, Richard Brightheart, M.Ac., L.Ac., L.M.P., has helped thousands of people recover their health by focusing on root-cause solutions. Many of his patients come to him with serious chronic debilitating illnesses. He has had excellent results with many of these patients by returning them back to a state of health. Rich incorporates a multitude of cutting edge therapies as well as specific nutritional and herbal support. He embraces the Chinese medicine model and meridian system. This system of energetic medicine is the body's core electromagnetic communication network, which is the basis for many of the modalities that Rich uses.

With such an in-depth educational background and a thorough understanding of anatomy and physiology from both Western and Eastern approaches, Rich has the unique ability to look beyond an individual's surface symptoms to see a much larger picture, which can identify the underlying causes of many illnesses. With his knowledge and diverse skills, he is able to break these puzzles down into smaller components, and has the ability and tools to reverse many of these conditions.

Rich received a master's degree in oriental medicine from the Northwest Institute of Oriental Medicine in Seattle, Washington, in 1998. He had previously studied sports medicine at University of Puget Sound in Tacoma, Washington. Rich has been licensed as a massage therapist since 1984. He holds dozens of educational certificates in many specialties that include: various forms of applied kinesiology (muscle testing), a full spectrum of energy medicine modalities, various Chinese meridian-based therapies, several soft tissue dysfunction/rehabilitation therapies, compromised immune and autoimmune-related illness, nutritional and environmental sensitivity repatterning, functional medicine, homeopathy, homotoxicology, herbal/nutritional support and detoxification. In addition to his formal education, Rich has spent thousands of hours of independent study in the fields of immunology, microbiology, biochemistry, pathology, autoimmune illnesses, emotional healing, allergies, detoxification, herbal medicine, nutritional support, energy medicine and soft tissue pain and dysfunction.

Rich has taught anatomy and physiology, structural and functional kinesiology, applied kinesiology and clinical injury rehabilitation and massage therapy at three massage schools and one kinesiology school. He was also co-owner of a massage therapy school.